*Stalking
the Healthful
Herbs*

Also by Euell Gibbons

Stalking the Wild Asparagus
Stalking the Blue-Eyed Scallop

Stalking the Healthful Herbs

by EUELL GIBBONS

with drawings of plants by
RAYMOND W. ROSE

Alan C. Hood & Company, Inc.

Chambersburg, Pennsylvania

Stalking the Healthful Herbs

Manufactured in the United States of America.

Library of Congress Cataloging-in-Publication Data

Gibbons, Euell.

Stalking the healthful herbs / Euell Gibbons ; with drawing of
plants by Raymond W. Rose.
    p.   cm:.
Reprint. Originally published: New York : D. McKay, 1966.
Includes index.
ISBN 0-911469-06-0
1. Herbs—United States.   2. Medicinal plants—United States.   3.
Wild plants, Edible—United States.   4. Herbs—Canada. 5. Medicinal
plants—Canada.   6. Wild plants, Edible—Canada.   7. Herbs--
Therapeutic use. 8. Herbs—Folklore.   9. Cookery (Wild foods) I. Title.
QK99.U6G53   1989
581.6'3—dc20
                                                    89-7617
                                                    CIP

Published by Alan C. Hood & Company, Inc.
Chambersburg, Pennsylvania

10 9 8 7

This book is dedicated to
the wonderful group of teenagers
who are members of the Future
Scientists Program of the Natural
Science Museum of Cleveland, Ohio,
and to
the Staff Coordinator of this inspired
educational project,
RUSSELL F. HANSEN

Acknowledgments

A NYONE who delves deeply into herbal lore will soon be in debt to writers who have been dead for hundreds, or even thousands, of years, for this is the most ancient of sciences. To Hippocrates and Theophrastus of ancient Greece, to Galen and Pliny of classic Rome, to those half-quack, half-genius herbalists of 17th-century England, Gerard and Culpepper, and to all the other many ancients whose herbal writings have survived, I owe much. True, these ancient writings contain much error, superstition, and arrant nonsense when examined in the light of modern science, but amazingly, there is also much solid fact and dependable information in these old books, and all of them, superstitious lore and all, have furnished me many months of fascinating reading, for which I am deeply grateful.

Among modern herbalists I am most indebted to Nelson Coon, author of *Using Plants for Healing*, and to Mrs. Maud Grieve of England, author of *A Modern Herbal*. If I have not always given these scholars the credit that is due them it is for the sake of brevity and style, and not because I do not realize the debt that I owe them.

I am particularly indebted to Dr. George Barron, Head of Foods and Nutrition in the Department of Home Economics at Pennsylvania State University, and to Mrs. Herta Lagally, Laboratory Technician, and her Student Assistant, Patricia Price, whose interest and help led to the discovery of unusual food values in many of the wild herbs mentioned in this book. Then there is Ray Rose, who not only made the line drawings that illustrate this work, but also spent many hours with me in field and kitchen, collecting and experimenting with strange forms of plant life. He boldly sampled many unusual remedies, beverages, confections, and outlandish concoctions without complaint. To all these kind people, and to the many others who helped to make this book a possibility, I am most grateful.

EUELL GIBBONS

Contents

Foreword

THE PLANTS that man has used throughout the ages as flavoring agents, medicines, and fragrances form a fascinating subject for study. (Many authorities now define an herb as any plant that was or is used for fragrance and scent, for culinary purposes, or for its healing properties, and also for its value as dye material.) From primitive times to the present day, man has employed such herbs to add to his comfort and well-being. In all parts of the world, native plants exist that possess or have been thought to possess virtues that appeal to the cook, the medicine man, and the witch doctor. Despite the fact that most wild herbs are of small economic importance in our modern civilization, nevertheless, they supply pleasure to an increasing number of people who study these plants and their fascinating lore.

The author of *Stalking the Healthful Herbs* brings to our attention in a delightful fashion many of the culinary and medicinal herbs native to North America—kinds that were well known to the Indians and early settlers. His intimate knowledge of these plants is based on countless field studies as well as on painstaking research. One clearly gets the feeling that he writes of what he knows and of what he has learned from endless experience and experiment.

—Elizabeth C. Hall
Associate Curator of Education,
The New York Botanical Garden
Honorary Member, New York Unit,
The Herb Society of America

Preface

I CANNOT TELL how my intense interest in nature began, for it was there as early as I can remember. At the age of five I originated my first wild food recipe, pounding together shelled hickory nuts and sweet hackberries to make a wild candy bar. My thirst for knowledge about nature was insatiable, and I picked the brains of every Indian, backwoodsman, and hillbilly I met. I had little formal schooling but became a gluttonous reader at an early age, and when not out in the fields and woods listening to what nature had to say, I was delving into books, learning what they had to teach about the wild things I loved.

While I was still a boy my parents moved to the hill country of New Mexico, and I became acquainted with the wild life of that arid region. I learned to forage for piñon nuts and became a connoisseur of cactus fruits. As soon as I was old enough to be on my own, I went to the Pacific Coast and began studying the exciting life forms and reveling in the gourmet food that could be gleaned from the edge of the sea. After several years on the West Coast, I went to Honolulu, where I attended the University of Hawaii, specializing in biology, botany, anthropology, and creative writing. I lived like a beachcomber, and much of my food was the wild tropical fruits I could gather in the mountains and the fish I caught from the sea.

There I met and married Freda, and a few years later we moved to Pennsylvania, my wife's native state, and I began the serious study of the flora and fauna of this richly endowed commonwealth. I was several years on the staff of Pendle Hill, a Quaker Graduate School at Wallingford, Pennsylvania. Since the school is in a semi-rural area, I continued my study of how wild things can be useful to man, and after leaving there, wrote two books, *Stalking the Wild Asparagus* and *Stalking the Blue-Eyed Scallop*, that tell how wild foods can be turned into gourmet delights.

We now live in an old Pennsylvania Dutch farmhouse near Beavertown, Pennsylvania, and have miles of uninhabited woodland on three sides of our place. We do not live on wild food, but we usually eat some wild foods every day. We don't feel there is special virtue in doing this—it is just that I love to gather and prepare these delicacies, and we like the taste of them. They are mere ornaments to our cuisine and have little effect on our food bill. We are not food faddists in any sense of the term.

We do often give dinners where every dish is made from wild ingredients, but this is frankly a stunt, and our guests are invariably enthusiastic about our wild parties. At a recent one, we served snapping-turtle soup, crayfish cocktail, tenderloin of venison in coconut-cream sauce, cattail bloom spikes cooked and served like asparagus, buttered milkweed buds, salad of wild watercress, sheep sorrel, purslane, and wild jerusalem artichokes, bread made of wild persimmons, and hickory nuts served with a wide assortment of wild fruit jams and jellies, sassafras tea, May-apple chiffon pie, and various other wild delicacies and nibbles thrown in at strategic points. We have also several times gone into wilderness areas and lived entirely on wild foods for as long as a week, and such outings always become continuous feasts, but I would not care to live that way all the time.

I have been accused of considering nature no more than a free larder from which to take gourmet food, but this is not true. My love affair with nature is so deep that I am not satisfied with being a mere onlooker, or nature tourist. I crave a more real and meaningful relationship. The spicy teas and tasty delicacies I prepare from wild ingredients are the bread and wine in which I have communion and fellowship with nature, and with the Author of that nature.

EUELL GIBBONS

Stalking
the Healthful
Herbs

1. Those Green Things

A GREEN BOOM is sweeping our land. Scientists and commercial drug producers are discovering that there is gold among the greens. Grandma's remedies, old wives' cures, folk medicine, and the teachings of the ancient herbalists are being reexamined today in scientific laboratories with the utmost seriousness. Even the layman has caught some of this fever, and those green things that grow by country waysides are being viewed as separate plants of hundreds of species, each having a unique structure and all presenting exciting possibilities of being useful to man.

It seems strange in this era of relatively sophisticated scientific knowledge, when man has probed the structure of the atom and can send a rocket to the moon, that we still do not know even the simple and easily determined chemical analyses of 95 percent of the common wild plants that spring up on every abandoned field or vacant lot. The science of chemurgic investigation of uncultivated plant life is still in its infancy. The vegetable kingdom remains virtually unexplored. Here is a tremendously promising area for researchers looking for new worlds to conquer; although it has barely been touched, it has already yielded great benefits to mankind. Often a single discovery opens up a whole new field.

For centuries, Greek shepherds dressed infected wounds with mold that grew on their bread when it was kept too long. Finally, a modern scientist looked at a culture of this mold (*Penicillium*) through a microscope. He not only discovered penicillin, but opened the door to the new science of antibiotics, which has brought to modern medicine some of its most potent healers. Now, other researchers are discovering that it is not only the simple molds and lowly fungi that produce these germ fighters, but that many of the higher plants, those neglected wild weeds that turn the countryside green every spring, also produce antibiotic substances that may soon be helping modern medicine in its battle against disease. (See page 212.)

Snakeroot, *Rauwolfia serpentina*, is a wild herb of India that has been used in the rich folk medicine of that country for thousands of years. An American researcher studied its use by native herbalists, then prevailed upon a Boston doctor to try it on patients suffering from high blood pressure. It not only lowered the dangerously high blood pressure of these patients, but the doctor noticed that after taking this medicine for a few days the patients became strangely calm, serene, and free from anxiety. He reported these benign side effects to psychiatrists, and this lowly plant, formerly a primitive herbal medicine, soon became a useful therapeutic agent in treating the mentally ill, and opened up the whole area of treatment with tranquilizers.

Curare is an arrow poison used by natives of South American jungles. Its active principle comes from an extract of a vine closely related to the moonseed (*Menispermum canadense*) of our local flora. Science examined this deadly substance and found that it killed by so relaxing the muscles that the animal could no longer stand or breathe. Carefully controlled doses of this usually lethal poison were found to relax the involuntary muscle spasms that accompany certain dread diseases of human beings. In laboratories, curare is now being broken down and many more of its secrets are being laid bare; as a result, a whole new line of antispasmodics is being developed, promising new hope to those afflicted with spastic paralysis and multiple sclerosis.

Often, in recent years, organized medicine, after disregarding a folk remedy or herbal medicine for decades, has discovered, either through investigation of the remedy in question, or—as more often happens—discovered through independent research, that the old wives were on the right track after all. Folk medicine has much wisdom in it, but still should not be swallowed whole. Any scientifically trained person who peruses the old herbals with a critical eye will soon discover that the gems of real truth, and the promising leads for research, are almost buried in obvious error, rank superstition, and transparent nonsense. This material must be put through the sieve of scientific method, if we are to extract the fraction of genuine knowledge and real benefits to mankind to be found there. Let the herbalist and the medical researcher work together, instead of at odds with one another, and we will see some startling progress in this field.

This book does not make the pretense of being a comprehensive herbal, giving all the known data on every plant that has ever been listed among the medicinal herbs. Such a book would run to many volumes and would be unutterably boring. The herbs and plants you will meet in this book were selected in the most arbitrary manner imaginable. Out of the hundreds of herbs and plants that I have collected and studied, and with which I have experimented, I have merely selected those that are common and widely available to most of us, the ones that I believe will be most interesting to you, as they have been to me.

Readers who encounter my work for the first time in this volume may be dismayed to find that I have omitted such obviously valuable and well-known herbs as calamus, poke, sassafras, May apple and sorrel, as well as many other wild herbs of known worth and long-standing use in home remedies. It was not that I loved these and other known herbs less but that I loved them first, and you will find their food and home-remedy possibilities thoroughly discussed in one or another of my earlier works, *Stalking the Wild Asparagus* and *Stalking the Blue-Eyed Scallop*. My three books are almost a trilogy —one might consider them three volumes of one work—and they are intended to be used together.

I have included both the ancient lore and the modern, scientific uses of the herbs that I discuss, but the main emphasis is on what *you* can do with these plants. This is a do-it-yourself herbal for those who are not satisfied merely to read about the wonders these plants can perform. And yet, I would be dismayed if I thought that any reader would be likely to substitute the remedies and recipes found in this book for needed professional medical care. I am not a doctor and cannot, nor do I wish to, prescribe for your ills. My attitude in this matter is probably best revealed by the fact that if I were to have a serious illness or injury I would immediately seek the services of a competent doctor rather than run to the woods for a medicinal herb.

However, home and herbal remedies still have a place in preventing and treating some of man's minor ills. Home remedies made of fresh herbs are often fully as effective as, and less dangerous than, many of the "patent" or proprietary medicines that are widely advertised and sold commercially. Most thinking doctors will admit that the home use of herbal remedies to stave off, or aid recovery from, minor ills and injuries is perfectly legitimate. A few years ago, Dr. Vincent Askey, then president of the American Medical Association, wrote an article for *This Week* magazine, deploring the growing belief that folk medicine and herbal remedies could substitute for scientific medical treatment. While expressing his reservations about trusting too strongly in herbal remedies, he admitted, "Home remedies probably always will have a place in the treatment of mankind's aches and pains. Physicians do not expect, and do not desire, that patients shall dash to the doctor with every minor discomfort, every trifling injury, every small ache or pain. It is sensible to care for such things by simple, safe home means."

This is my position exactly, except that there is more to be said. When you read further, you will notice that I recommend many of the flavorful and fragrant herbs and plants discussed in this book as food and drink for the well, rather than as medicine for the sick. It is a point hard to prove, but I believe the regular use of these wild plants, not as medicine, but as part of the daily diet, has some prophylactic, or preventive, value in warding off illness. I am firmly convinced that if we made more use of these fresh green herbs and plants, with their high vitamin and mineral contents, we would need to impose on the time of the physician far less often than we now do.

I am not a gardener or farmer, but a wanderer in remote places and byways, so I limit myself to the plants that grow wild and avoid domestic herbs. I am not even interested in bringing wild plants under cultivation; indeed, in a few cases, as with sage and horehound, I will tell you how to make tame plants go wild. It is not that I have anything against herb gardening; it is probably a fascinating hobby, but it doesn't happen to be mine. The plants I love are the wild ones, and for my part they can stay that way. Raising rabbits and pheasants is no real substitute for hunting, and raising fish in a pond is not an adequate alternative to going fishing. I love the search for these wild plants, and thrill in finding and collecting them from their native habitats. Forcing them to grow in neat orderly rows would remove half the meaning from the game.

The wild herbs I love came to me one by one, and that is the way I present them to you. In most cases, I first met them in the pages of an old herbal, or in the journal of an early naturalist. Or, it may have been in a scientific paper on the ethnobotany of some Amerindian tribe. Such literature forms my bedtime reading. When some plant seems to stand out as especially interesting, useful, or otherwise desirable, I search out all references to it in other herbal literature. A search through a good medical library tells me what modern science is doing, if anything, with this same plant. All this gives me much information and lore about the plant, but it is secondhand knowledge, and my eyes want to see, my tongue to taste, my nose to smell, and my fingers to handle, this plant. This is the spirit that drives me into the wilderness.

Botanical drugs from herbal suppliers, or herbarium specimens of these plants, will not do. Trying to determine the nature of living plants from these mummified remains is like trying to study the nature of man in a morgue. I must go into the wilds and find the living plant. When I finally discover a long-sought plant, I always experience a thrill of pleasure and gratitude. I understand the feelings of those old Indian medicine men, who, when seeking medicinal herbs, would not pluck the first specimen found, but would sit down by it, bury a little tobacco by its roots as a thank offering, then meditate awhile and go on until they found other plants of the same species to collect and use. They believed that finding an abundant supply of the herb they were seeking depended upon faithfully following this ritual with the first specimen encountered. This was not the unreasoning superstition that it sounds, and I have found they were right.

Meditating on the first specimen of a plant that is new to me opens my eyes and sharpens my awareness until other plants of the same species become visible, standing out from the green background in an abundance that was always there, but which I was unprepared to see until I had gazed deeply at a single specimen. When I collect such plants, take them into my kitchen, and transform them with my own hands into some fragrant or savory seasoning, a delicious dish, or a benign remedy, it has a totally different meaning from using a commercial product. A remedy in which both nature and I have entered deeply does something for my soul as well as for my body.

I know there are people for whom wild plants don't invoke the same kind of response that **they** do in me. Some are merely indifferent—they couldn't care less whether those green things have values they could use or not—but others are actively antipathetic to the whole notion of making friends with these wildings. They are a little frightened by a plant that grows where man did not will it to grow, indeed where he may have tried to eradicate it. We spray our roadsides with deadly herbicides, giving them the appearance of having been struck by an ugly blight; we rip out the natural growth and replace it with familiar and "safe" domestic plants; we clear away the thickets, mow the open places, level off the hills, and fill the swamps, without ever asking the name or nature of the plants that we are destroying.

There are those who think that the history of civilization is the story of man's conquest of nature, and they are not about to make friends with the untamed and unconquered remnants of the ancient enemy. Our artificial environment causes a one-sided development. If we live only on our civilized side, then contact with untamed nature becomes traumatic. It arouses a feeling of insecurity, and we rush with relief to a man-controlled environment. We become so dependent on the comfort and security of our artificial world that the continued existence of wild things, not under the ordering of man, seems a threat. We retaliate against this wild flora by name-calling, labeling it "weeds," "brush," or "briers."

The thought of really getting acquainted with wild plants, eating them, and taking them as medicine arouses an unconscious, primitive fear in some people, or a primitive fascination. Even in modern civilized man there is buried an element that is atavistic and untamed. We will never be whole men until we have learned to accept, and even to love, these primitive aspects of ourselves, and to see their counterparts and their fulfillment in the elements of nature itself that grow with no aid from the hand of man.

2. What's an Herb to Do With?

THE WAY young children define things by function always amuses me. I was out in the fields with my four-year-old nephew when a crow in a nearby thicket set up a raucous cawing and scolding. The little boy was slightly alarmed and asked, "What is that awful noise?" I told him it was a crow, and his fear turned to interest. His next question could have been foreseen by anyone who has ever studied children closely. He said, "Uncle Euell, what is a crow to do with?"

I, too, want to know what things are to do with. I have a deep and abiding love for nature, but unlike most nature-lovers, I am not content merely to look on. I have never felt alien to nature, and I resent allusions to mankind's "conquest of nature," for nature is my mother and I am her favorite child. Even when nature seems brutal or punishing, it is usually a just chastisement because we have willfully or ignorantly disobeyed some of her immutable laws. I seek out nature, not just to sightsee, but to "get with it." I am not even satisfied by collecting and identifying botanical specimens, for my curiosity extends far beyond the mere name and classification of each plant. Emerson said that a weed is "a plant whose virtues have not yet been discovered," and as I look at each unfamiliar plant with which I come in contact, I wonder how it can be useful to me, or add to my enjoyment of life. I want to know not only its size, shape, color, habits, and Latin name, but also its hidden constituents. What are its medicinal properties, and can it help me to heal my own aches and pains? Does it have a delightful odor, and can I use this scent in perfumes, sachets, potpourri jars, or to give an appetizing aroma to my food and drink? Above all, can I eat it, make a beverage of it, or use it to flavor my food and get an esoteric taste thrill that cannot be purchased in the marketplace? It is in such bread and wine that I find the deepest communion with nature.

An herb is to hunt. I seldom pick a strange plant, take it to my study, dissect its flower, note its features, then look it up in the appropriate manual, and finally start studying its constituents and virtues. I usually work the puzzle from the other end. No dedicated hunter goes out searching for birds and mammals at random, then turns to identifying the species he has shot, and I treat plants the same way. I first learn something about an herb, study descriptions and illustrations, memorize its identification features, learn something about its values and uses, then set out to find it in its native habitat. This way I am looking for a friend instead of a stranger, and experience a thrill of accomplishment when I finally track it down. This is an outdoor sport closely related to hunting and fishing, but without the gut-wringing twinges of conscience that always come to haunt me when I kill an innocent animal.

An herb is to learn. One acquires many new skills and a vast store of interesting knowledge in stalking the helpful herbs. The eye learns to detect small differences that went unnoticed before. The nose is trained to recognize hundreds of different aromas, and is then able to bring us a new awareness of the world about us. The taste is trained to recognize hundreds of subtle flavors for which we do not even have names. One learns how the close study of one plant can teach us a great deal about the whole plant kingdom. There is the exciting discovery that nature is not the chaos that it seems to the uninitiated, but has a marvelous order and harmony that lead to understandable classification. One learns to recognize relationships among plants, and then even the total stranger becomes partly known and loved. One finds that certain American plants show close relationship to other plants in far-off Asia or Africa, even though their ancestors have now been separated for millions of years. One begins to recognize the relationship of the wild rose to the wild cherry, and learns why such dissimilar plants as the May apple and the barberry are considered relatives, and why the skunk cabbage and the Jack-in-the-pulpit are said to be akin. Such knowledge gives new meaning to every wild plant we encounter.

An herb is to see. Or, as my Pennsylvania Dutch neighbors would put it, "A plant is for pretty." Everyone appreciates the conspicuous and flamboyant beauty of the larger wildflowers, but how many have thrilled to the sheer beauty of the thrice-pinnate foliage of the common yarrow that grows by every roadside? How many have ever seen the intricate beauty of the many wildflowers that are so tiny they must be studied under a magnifying glass? Once the eye is trained to see these things, one finds that nature has surrounded us with breathtaking beauty that largely goes unobserved and unappreciated.

An herb is to pick, to gather, to use. Here, some misguided nature-lovers and uninformed conservationists might take issue with me, but I am ready to defend my position. It is a serious mistake to equate conservation with non-use. Too often non-use leads to noninterest which leads to non-knowing or only partial acquaintance, and in this ignorance great destruction is wrought. Sometimes it is the conservationists who want to eradicate certain plants for which they can see no immediate use, even though they might have a thousand virtues of which they never dreamed. It is the forager, the lover of wild foods and the culler of herbs and simples who is most interested in the protection and preservation of these products of untamed nature, and he will learn to gather and use without destroying. He will not only know when and how to pick and use, but when to refrain from picking, so these simple wayside plants can be preserved for future generations to experience the joys they offer; sometimes an herb is to leave alone.

An herb is to taste. A great many of the wild plants have delightful flavors that can add new interest to salads, confections or other culinary preparations, lifting them from the humdrum class to that of gourmet products. Food should never be merely nourishment, a means of keeping us alive, but should be one of the amenities that make life a joy. The sheer enjoyment of food contributes to its digestibility and healthfulness, and a great many wild herbs have delicious and appropriate flavors that they stand ready to contribute—free—to this cause.

An herb is to smell. Most people know that many wildflowers have sweet and pleasant odors, but how many know that many wild plants also have fruit, foliage, and even roots, that exude delightful perfume? These joyful scents can not only be enjoyed out in the fields and woods, but can be captured in various ways to perfume our houses, clothes, and bodies, giving them the sweet, clean aromas of nature, rather than the cloying and powerful scents of the perfumers' art. Delightful smells not only give present enjoyment, but have a subtle effect on memory, and to introduce a child to the woodland odors is to give him the ability, in later years, to recapture the joys of childhood merely by smelling of a wild plant or fruit or a crushed leaf.

An herb is to cure our illnesses. There is simply no doubt that many herbs have weapons they stand ready to contribute to mankind's battle against disease and sickness. Although most of these will be administered by professional doctors, the home remedy has always been with us, and in some areas is here to stay. I know that home preparations can contribute to my comfort during certain minor illnesses and can relieve my minor aches and pains. Such home remedies have a further value in enabling the well members of the family to express their concern and love for the sick person by gathering and preparing a wild herb remedy and tenderly administering it to the patient. Such things also have value.

An herb is to eat. Some wild herbs successfully make the leap from mere condiments to hearty foods that can be served in ample helpings, and many of these are better vegetables than some that come regularly to our tables from commercial markets. The health benefits of herbs can often be better utilized and assimilated if the herb is eaten as food rather than taken as medicine, and some of these wild herbs are delicious. Wild plants can contribute variety and many new and delightful flavors to our diets.

An herb is to nourish our bodies. I had long suspected that a great many of the astonishing cures attributed to herbal medicines by the ancient practitioners of this art were due neither to magic nor to medicinal properties, but to the vitamins, minerals, and other nutrients contained in these plants. When one reads that an herb will cure such diverse complaints as poor vision; dull or inflamed and itching eyes; styes; pimples on the face; blackheads; dry, rough, and itching skin; boils and carbuncles; dull hair and dandruff; dry, rough throat; superficial tubercles about the neck and throat; cysts; and many kinds of infections, one is apt to dismiss such claims as nonsense, or to ascribe the results to psychological effect on the patient. But look again. All these complaints, thought of as different illnesses by the ancient herbalists, could be symptoms arising from a single cause, an acute deficiency of vitamin A.

Similarly, when one reads that a certain herb or plant will cure scurvy, poisoning, all manner of infections, pink toothbrush, and the tendency to bruise easily, and will even aid in healing battle wounds and broken bones, one suspects that what the plant really will do is correct a vitamin C shortage. Often, I have seen the above lists of complaints and herbal or plant cures combined, giving a clue that here are wild things rich in both vitamins A and C.

I approached the Food and Nutrition Department of Pennsylvania State University with this idea, and they became interested. We searched the literature and found that quite a number of the wild plants most commonly used as food had been thoroughly explored for their nutritional properties. We assembled this data and then plunged into the unknown. Because of limited time, personnel, and funds, our research project was necessarily small in scope and modest in its goals. By kitchen research I had determined that certain unusual and nutritionally unexplored plants were eminently edible, so we limited ourselves to finding the vitamin A and C content of these, with a few side excursions into their mineral and protein contents. I gathered the material and delivered it to the University, and a staff lab technician made the analyses. Even this almost superficial examination of only a few herbs yielded some exciting results and opened a field of great promise to some future and more ambitious researcher. We found that a small helping of cooked violet leaves, which are delicious when prepared and served like spinach, could furnish all one's daily minimum requirements of vitamins A and C, and are probably good sources of other nutrients. Even violet flowers were found to be a good food, rich in protective vitamins. The common nettle, a favorite potherb of many foragers, not only proved an excellent source of vitamins A and C, but also is exceedingly rich in protein. Wild mint, besides its ability to contribute an almost universally liked flavor and fragrance, proved to be very rich in vitamins A and C, and should be eaten—not merely used as a seasoning and garnish.

After engaging in this research, I understood why the children of my Pennsylvania Dutch neighbors ate violet blossoms and chewed on catnip and mint. Their wise little bodies were informing these children what was needed. I also understood how they could maintain glowing health on a seemingly inadequate diet. They were getting their vitamins, minerals, and other food supplements from the wild plants they were consuming between meals. If we are ever cut off from our present sources of fresh food and diet supplements, we need never suffer from malnutrition if only we know which wild plants to reach for. The malnourished poor of some depressed rural areas could achieve glowing and abundant health, if only one could persuade them to eat the vitamin-rich wild plants that grow all about them.

And finally, an herb is to enjoy. Exploring the possible uses of wild plants has furnished me with a fascinating, lifelong hobby that has brought me more hours of pleasant recreation than anything else on God's green earth. I have found that children are easily interested in this sport and when properly guided will spend many pleasant and highly educational hours in pursuit of knowledge about wild vegetation. A child will probably be bored stiff by any attempt to teach him formal botany, but the whole picture changes when he knows what a plant is to do with. Anyone who plunges into this hobby with diligence and enthusiasm will soon learn that an herb is to love.

3. Wild Horseradish as Medicine, Condiment, and Cosmetic

(*Armoracia lapathifolia*)

EVERYONE knows that horseradish is a biting condiment that adds zest to boiled beef, venison, smoked tongue, or raw oysters, but a lot of us are not also aware that horseradish is a common wild plant in this country and it has become abundantly naturalized in low meadows and along ditches. Although no doubt originally introduced as a garden plant, horseradish is able to maintain itself in the wild, and early escaped from domestication. It still seems to prefer the vicinity of man, however, and one seldom finds wild horseradish in a remote wilderness.

Horseradish is a perennial with cylindrical, almost conical white roots often more than a foot long and up to two inches in diameter, abruptly branched at the lower ends. Any one of these small root branches is capable of producing a new plant, making the horseradish extremely persistent once it is established. You don't have to feel like a vandal when digging wild horseradish, for there is no danger of exterminating it, and once a patch of this wild vegetable is located, you can return to the same patch year after year to harvest a supply. The removal of the old roots and the digging you do will merely encourage it and make it grow more luxuriantly than ever.

As you might guess from its flavor, this plant is a member of the mustard family, but its leaves do not betray this relationship to the untrained eye. A majority of the leaves spring directly from the top of the root, and are on long, stout, channeled leafstalks. The leaf blade is dark green, about a foot long and five inches wide, with wavy edges and widespreading teeth. When the flower stalk springs up, it bears small, oblong, unstalked leaves that are sharply toothed. The flowers are borne in panicles and are small and white. Like other members of the mustard family, each flower has four petals, arranged in the shape of a cross, with six stamens, four long and two short.

The roots can be dug any time of the year that the ground is not frozen. If a supply of roots is gathered in late autumn and stored in wet sand in a cool cellar, they will keep until new roots can be gathered in the spring. To make the common condiment called prepared horseradish, select firm, white, crisp, roots, grate them fine, and add enough vinegar to make it the consistency of a custard. Strangely, the hot, biting taste and pungent aroma do not exist in the unbroken root, but are developed during the grating by a chemical reaction between constituents that are found in separate cells in the growing plant. Therefore, horseradish has to be grated fine before it has much flavor. If you want to preserve its hotness keep prepared horseradish in the refrigerator.

An easy way to grate horseradish is in an electric blender. Simply put 1 cup of diced horseradish root and ¼ cup of vinegar in the blender and run at high speed for about 3 minutes. For use on boiled beef or boiled tongue, leave it plain. If it is to be used on pork, mix 1 tablespoonful of ground dry mustard with each batch. An unusual and exceedingly tasty horseradish can be made by adding a teaspoonful of crushed dill seed to a cup of prepared horseradish. To get still other flavors, and to enjoy new taste thrills, substitute aniseed or oregano for the dill. If you would like to tame the fierce pungency of wild horseradish and at the same time give it an attractive red color, mix together in a blender ½ cup of diced horseradish, ½ cup of diced red beets, ¼ cup of cider vinegar, and a teaspoon of dill seed. Some like to add a teaspoon of honey to this mixture. This makes a mild condiment that goes well with most meats; guests of ours who thought they didn't like horseradish have raved about this mixture.

Horseradish has a venerable history. There is little doubt that this was the plant called *Raphanos agrios*, or wild radish, by the ancient

Greeks. It is said to be one of the five bitter herbs the Jews were commanded to eat at the Passover meal with cooked lamb and unleavened bread. This was apparently originally intended as a discipline, or asceticism, but I really can't feel very sorry for a people who have been commanded to eat boiled lamb with horseradish and matzos. It makes me hungry merely to write about it. Nor do the other four "bitter herbs"—coriander, lettuce, horehound, and nettle—inspire much sympathy for a people who had to eat them. I often eat all five purely for pleasure.

To the knowledgeable forager, the lowly wild horseradish is much more than a mere relish to eat with meat or seafood. The first leaves that spring up from the crown of the horseradish, gathered when young and tender, are some of the finest salad greens and boiling greens to be found in the wild, with a flavor resembling that of watercress. Such a mundane food as a liverwurst sandwich becomes a gourmet item when the liverwurst is spread on buttered hot rye toast and garnished with a few newly born leaves of horseradish. A few of these same tender leaves chopped fairly fine can add distinction and robust character to what would otherwise be a very ordinary tossed salad.

As a cooked vegetable, horseradish leaves are too emphatic when used alone; more palates will be pleased when they are mixed with milder, blander greens. My own favorite plant to blend with horseradish greens is another of those ancient Jewish "bitter herbs," the nettle. Young, tender nettles and the first leaves of the horseradish usually appear at about the same time of year, and are often found growing near one another, for both require the same kinds of moisture and soil conditions. Gather equal quantities of nettle tops and horseradish leaves, or a little more of the nettles. Wash the greens together, stirring them in the wash water with a stick or long-handled spoon to avoid coming in contact with the stinging cells of the nettles. Lift them from the wash water directly into the cooking pot, using kitchen tongs or a perforated spoon. The water that clings to the freshly washed leaves is all the cooking water they need. Cook gently for about 20 minutes, then chop them right in the pot, using a hefty pair of kitchen shears for this operation. Season with butter or bacon fat, a little salt, and a sprinkle of cider vinegar, and serve.

Even with this almost waterless cooking method, there will still be some juice in the pot. Don't drain it off or throw it away, for this liquid is a potent nutrient concentrate, rich in vitamins A and C and many of the trace minerals essential to glowing health. Either serve the juice with the greens or drink it. I like a bowl of this "potlikker" with some buttered corn bread that has been baked in thin, crusty pones and served hot from the oven.

Strangely, except for that one mention of horseradish in Jewish law cited above, we do not find a single reference to horseradish as a food or condiment in ancient literature. The ancients were familiar with the plant, but they apparently thought of it only as a medicinal herb. Those lusty gourmets, the ancient Greeks and Romans, never knew the joys of horseradish on their meats and seafoods. Pliny, writing in the 1st century, praises its curative powers, but fails to mention any food or condiment uses of horseradish. In the rich herbal literature of the British Isles there are references to horseradish as a valuable medicinal plant, going back to the 13th century, but it was not thought of as comestible until much later. In the late 16th century one herbalist finally mentions its use by the Germans "as a sauce to eate fish with and such like meates as we do mustarde," but it is not until 1640 that a writer mentions its use as a condiment in England, and he damns it with faint praise, writing that it is used only by "country people and strong laboring men," and adding "it is too strong for tender and gentle stomachs." Not long after, however, horseradish did begin appearing on the tables of the gentry.

As a medicinal herb, both the root and the leaves of horseradish have long been recommended as efficacious in curing many illnesses. It seemed a habit of ancient herbalists to claim that almost any herb being written about would cure just about any illness to which human beings are subject. Such multiple claims are more reasonably made for horseradish than for almost any other herb. Horseradish therapy has stood the test of time and is still widely used in home remedies, and horseradish preparations still appear in some pharmacopoeias. It is classed as stimulant, rubefacient, diuretic, antiscorbutic, diaphoretic, vermifuge, and expectorant.

Horseradish is reputed to be a strong and active diuretic, and even modern writers have claimed that it will prevent kidney stones if eaten regularly, and even expel stones already formed, if taken before they grow too large. For the same reason, it has been used to treat dropsy when the fluid accumulations are caused by too scanty a flow of urine. Horseradish is said to prevent infestations of parasitical intestinal worms and to expel them when already present. Horseradish root contains more vitamin C than lettuce or green peppers, and was formerly an important antiscorbutic, chiefly because it could be obtained in winter, when the common vitamin-deficient diet of dried and salted foods caused scurvy to become a plague. In treatment of the common cold, horseradish can fortify the body with vitamin C, promote perspiration, stimulate the nerves, loosen phlegm and congestion, and relieve sore throat, hoarseness, and coughing. It probably never cures a cold, but then, neither do any of the widely advertised and expensive cold medicines sold on the market. Horseradish is a stimulant to the appetite and a spur to a languid digestion. All these benefits can be had, not by taking it as a medicine, but merely by eating it as a tasty relish on meats or seafood.

Grated horseradish has also been used externally, replacing the more drastic mustard plaster. Here it acts as a stimulant and rubefacient, drawing blood to the area and reddening the skin. One old herbalist writes, "If bruised and laid on a part grieved with sciatica, gout, joint-ache or hard swellings of the spleen and liver, it doth wonderfully help them all." A fairly modern work makes the following almost unbelievable statement, "For facial neuralgia, some of the fresh scrapings (of horseradish) if held in the hand on the affected side, will give relief—the hand in some cases within a short time becoming bloodlessly white and benumbed." I fail to see how a medicine held in the hand can affect a pain in the face, and I also cannot see how a substance that will cause reddening of the skin on other parts of the body can cause the hand to turn white and become bloodless. I don't have enough faith in this remedy even to try it, but then, I am not suffering from neuralgia. A more reasonable external use of horseradish is as a poultice to treat chilblains and mild frostbites. Here its rubefacient properties would no doubt hasten the healing of the circulatory system that has been damaged by frost or cold by attracting more healing blood to that area.

Besides protecting my health by freely using horseradish as a relish or in a seafood cocktail sauce, and eating horseradish salads and greens in the spring, I also make some home remedies from this versatile plant. One winter a houseguest came down with influenza, and an old herbal book I owned recommended a wine infusion of horseradish for this malady. The directions were very indefinite about quantities and dosage, so I made the infusion by the trial-and-taste method, which resulted in my getting a prophylactic overdose of this influenza remedy. The proportions I finally settled on were 2 tablespoons of prepared horseradish, 2 tablespoons of honey, a dash of nutmeg, and a twist of orange peel, all stirred into a pint of claret wine that had been heated to 160° in the top of a double boiler. This was given to the patient as hot as he could drink it, a wineglassful at a time, four times a day. After the first dose, the wine was reheated in the double boiler each time it was to be given.

I also called in a doctor, and while he was there I questioned whether he approved of my remedy. He wanted to taste the mixture, so we went to the kitchen and made up a fresh batch. It is not the gruesome glop it sounds like, and is surprisingly palatable. He sampled it, smacked his lips, and passed his glass back for more. When the pint was finished, and he began to bundle up in overcoat and muffler to brave the cold, he said, "I don't know whether that remedy will do anything for the patient or not, but it has certainly done wonders for me."

When I have a heavy lecture schedule, or when I just talk too much, I sometimes get hoarse. When this happens, I add 1 tablespoon of vinegar and 2 tablespoons of grated horseradish to ⅓ cup of water and allow it to infuse for about 1 hour. Then I carefully pour the liquid off the settled horseradish, and to the liquid I add ⅔ cup of honey. I take a teaspoonful of this mixture every hour until my hoarseness is gone. This remedy contains no dangerous drugs, and it, too, is surprisingly palatable. Children take it eagerly, and it can safely be given to them.

Although beauty treatments are a hopeless waste of effort in my case, I was interested to learn that horseradish has been widely used in cosmetics for skin that lacks clearness or freshness. One herbalist recommends soaking 1 part horseradish in 4 parts fresh milk for 1 hour, then using the milk as a skin freshener. This source also claims that this milk-and-horseradish mixture will cure itch and other skin troubles. Among the many trace minerals found in horseradish there is a large percentage of sulfur, and this might account for its efficacy as a skin freshener and healer of minor skin disorders. I actually made some of this mixture and tried it, not with any hope of becoming beautiful, but because I wanted to be sure it would not take the skin off the face of some beauty. I used it as an after-shave lotion, but found I disliked the feeling of milk drying on my face.

Trying to improve on this formula, I experimented, combining two good cosmetic herbs, horseradish and witch-hazel. The proportions that seem to work best are: to 2 cups of distilled witch-hazel water add ½ cup of grated horseradish and allow it to meld overnight, then strain and discard the spent horseradish. To this liquid add ½ cup of commercial rubbing alcohol and ¼ cup of white vinegar. This makes a lively and effective skin bracer, and my wife says she likes it better than any commercial skin freshener obtainable. When I complained that the aroma of horseradish and vinegar made her face and hands smell like a well-dressed salad, she added some cologne to the formula, to the great improvement of its fragrance, After that I tried it as an after-shave lotion, and liked it.

Whether used as food or as a cosmetic, horseradish should never be cooked. Heat dispels its sprightly piquancy and leaves it tasting like a very poor grade of cooked turnips; I don't know a worse thing that I could say about any food.

PEPPERROOT, CROW'S-FOOT, OR WILD HORSERADISH
(*Dentaria laciniata*)

Did you ever eat boiled buffalo tongue with horseradish? I did, and I'm not that old, either. This tongue was from a ranch-raised and grain-fattened buffalo (bison) that had been purchased by a butcher who was selling the meat at fancy prices. I didn't pay the fancy prices, either; I merely wangled an invitation to have dinner at the butcher's home, which wasn't hard to do, as I was courting his daughter. When I enter a butcher shop today and see the prices they are getting for meat, I sometimes wish I had married her.

As we were enjoying our unusual meal, her younger brother asked me if the Indians ate horseradish with buffalo meat. I sometimes suspect this boy liked me better than his sister ever did, for he could be depended on to steer the conversation into channels where I was most knowledgeable, bless him. I explained that horseradish was a naturalized plant, introduced by the early settlers, and therefore could not have been known to the Indians before the coming of the white man. This little boy had been a bit disappointed to discover that buffalo meat, to which he had looked forward with avid anticipation, had turned out to be little, if any, better than ordinary beef. He had found that the only way he liked this overrated delicacy was to disguise it with condiments, so he asked, "If they didn't have

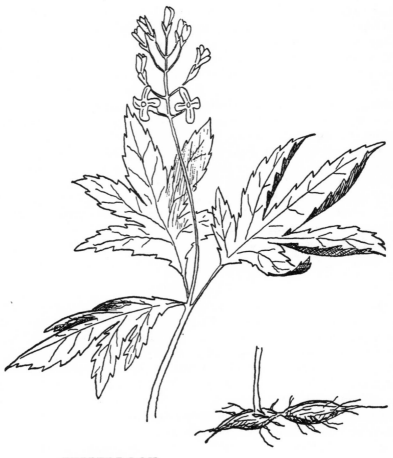

PEPPERROOT

horseradish, what did they put on buffalo meat to make it taste good?"

Although the Indians didn't have horseradish, they did have a passable substitute in a native plant called pepperroot, actually a relative of the real horseradish, that grows in wooded areas throughout the eastern half of our country from Maine to Minnesota and south to Florida and Louisiana. It is a small plant, seldom more than a foot high, and is one of the common spring flowers, appearing, in Pennsylvania, in March and April. Each plant is but a single thin stem bearing three stalked leaves arranged in a whorl just below the flower panicle. Each leaf is deeply cut into three linear segments, the divisions toothed at the margins. This three-part leaf has caused the plant to be called crow's-foot in some sections, although it is unrelated to the true crowfoot family. Like the horseradish, this plant belongs to the mustard family, but the relationship is not readily discovered unless one examines the blossoms or tastes the root. The blossoms are borne on a panicle, the lower ones opening first, and they, like most members of the mustard family, have four petals arranged in the shape of a cross, and six stamens, four of them long and two of them shorter. The blossoms are about three-fourths of an inch across, white to purple-pink in color, and rather attractive. The edible root consists of a series of oval joints, from a half-inch to an inch long, strung together like a necklace, the joints freely separating.

Gathering these roots in quantity would be a tedious job, but one seldom wants many of them. They are more a condiment than a food. When I am hiking in wooded country in the early spring, I often dig a few to eat with my sandwiches. The flavor is the same pungent, mustardy taste one finds in horseradish. I have grated and pounded pepperroot with a little vinegar to make a camp horseradish, but it should be eaten in camp, for when one eats it in a dining room with butcher's meats and an indoor appetite, one discovers that it isn't really as good as horseradish.

There are four or five other species of *Dentaria* (botanists disagree on the exact number) growing in this country, but after becoming familiar with one species you will find the other species similar enough to be recognizable. All of them have peppery roots that are wholesome and flavorful when used as condiments. I have never heard of any medicinal use of the pepperroots, but they are pretty little plants, well worth knowing, and the pungent roots can make an otherwise uninteresting sandwich something to remember.

4. Witch-Hazel:

MOST FAMILIAR OF ALL
HERBAL MEDICINES

(Hamamelis virginiana)

WITCH-HAZEL is probably better known and more widely used than any other herbal remedy. The first settlers learned of its manifold uses from the Indians, and it soon came to be considered a household necessity, a position it holds to this day. Although the distilled extract of witch-hazel can be found on most bathroom shelves, there are many who do not realize that this well-known remedy is made from a familiar shrub that they have probably seen a thousand times. Witch-hazel is a very common bush or small tree from Maine to Florida and west to the Plains. Several small trunks usually spring from one root, and the whole shrub may reach a height of 10 to 12 feet. It is found in rich woods and along little streams. The leaves are three to five inches long and a little more than half that wide, oval in shape, with wavy, toothed margins, downy when young. This plant reverses the usual order of things by blooming in the fall, just after it sheds its leaves. The blossoms are small and yellow, each having four slender strap-shaped petals. For use in home remedies, the leaves are gathered when full-grown and spread in a warm place to dry. The distilled extract is usually made of the twigs, which should be cut in winter while the shrub is dormant.

Witch-hazel is listed as having astringent, tonic, sedative, and hemostatic properties, and it has been used in poultices, infusions, decoctions, ointments, suppositories, fluidextracts, and distilled extracts, as a powdered drug, and in cosmetics. It has been recom-

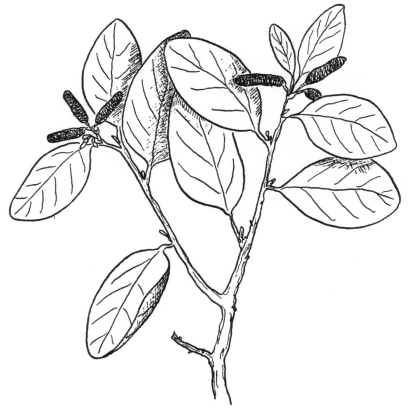

WITCH-HAZEL

mended for treating internal and external hemorrhage, bruises, inflammation, hemorrhoids, diarrhea, dysentery, varicose veins, burns,
scalds, insect bites, and bags under the eyes. If these uses are superstitious, as some claim, they are superstitions that are shared in high
places, for witch-hazel is an official drug in the U.S. *Pharmacopoeia,*
the *National Formulary,* and the *U.S. Dispensatory.* And yet, despite
all these recommendations, there is far from being complete agree-
ment in the medical profession as to its uses and efficacy. Some
maintain that none of its present uses can be scientifically justified
and consider this long-established botanical drug inert and useless.

Useless or not, the public obviously intends to keep on using it, for about one million gallons of distilled witch-hazel extract is produced and sold every year. The householders who buy and use this vast river of witch-hazel feel that it *does* help in healing minor complaints, whether or not scientists can explain how or why it helps. I consider witch-hazel the very epitome of all that a herbal remedy intended for home use should be. It is harmless and perfectly safe to use and mild and gentle in action. This is no wonder drug, or miracle cure, with drastic and dramatic effects. As I see the role of witch-hazel in home remedies, it is to give a little help in correcting certain malfunctions, some minor aid in helping the body to repair its own breakdowns, and some little relief from the discomforts of minor complaints, while nature, the greatest doctor of them all, brings the system back into top working order.

I have a friend, a little girl, who is intensely interested in wild foods and herbal remedies. Once we stood before a witch-hazel bush while I explained its reputed therapeutic uses, the controversy over them, and my own ideas on the subject. At the end of a half-hour lecture she brilliantly summarized all I had said by remarking, "As I understand it, witch-hazel will help nearly everything, but not very much." There you have it! Witch-hazel is useful in a large number of minor complaints, but its action is likely to be gently corrective and unspectacular.

The constituents of witch-hazel are not impressive; it contains tannic and gallic acids, as do many plants used in home remedies, an unidentified bitter principle, and a small amount of volatile oil. You can make your own distilled Witch-Hazel Extract by using the drip still shown on page 167, but I doubt that many will wish to do so, as commercial witch-hazel extract is almost universally available and inexpensive. If you insist on making your own, as I did, gather 2 pounds of dormant witch-hazel twigs. Cut these in lengths not over ½ inch. Put the chopped twigs in your blender with 8 cups of water (in two batches, if your blender is a small one) and blend until the witch-hazel is cut very fine. Allow the blended twigs to soak in this same water overnight. Next day pour twigs and water into the drip still, put it on very high heat, and collect 2 cups of distillate, then discard the spent material left in the still. To the 2 cups of distillate add ½ cup of rubbing alcohol; bottle the extract, and it is ready to use. I added pure grain alcohol on which I had to pay the Pennsylvania beverage-alcohol tax and found my homemade extract cost considerably more than I would have had to pay for ready-made witch-hazel of standard U.S.P. grade at the druggist's.

When people say "witch-hazel" in referring to medicine, they usually mean this distilled extract to which about 15 percent of alcohol has been added, so it will not spoil. It has many uses. Because of its tannin content, it is an excellent first-aid treatment for minor burns and scalds. Dabbed on the skin with a cotton pad, it will soothe insect stings and mosquito bites. Witch-hazel is supposed to have a strengthening effect on the muscular fiber of veins. A fine first-aid treatment for burst varicose veins is to wet a compress with witch-hazel extract and tape it tightly to the burst vein. This will stop the bleeding and may prevent serious loss of blood when medical help is long in coming.

Most women already know how to use witch-hazel extract in preserving their youth and beauty. Its astringency makes it an excellent skin freshener, and a safe treatment for many minor skin blemishes. If you are feeling overworked and under-loved, nervous and irritable, and your mirror tells you that bags are beginning to form under your eyes, drop everything, forget your worries, lie down and put two cotton pads soaked in witch-hazel over your eyes and think nothing but beautiful thoughts for at least 15 minutes. You can buy sterilized eye-shaped cotton pads made especially for this purpose. You will find this one of the finest, most effective, and least expensive of all beauty treatments.

The Iroquois Indians formerly made a tea-like beverage of dried witch-hazel leaves, which they sweetened with maple sugar. I tried making this tea using about the same amount of witch-hazel leaves as I would use of ordinary tea, and it was not bad, having a somewhat austere flavor and roughening the tongue like overstrong tea. A little milk tamed it down considerably, and it would make an acceptable camp tea whenever the imported product is not available. Unsweetened, this tea becomes an efficacious remedy for diarrhea and dysentery, where its tannic astringency is put to good use. Its tannin content also makes this tea, when cooled, an excellent gargle for sore throat, but make it fresh often, as it is likely to spoil if kept for several days.

A strong infusion made of half an ounce of dried witch-hazel leaves to a pint of boiling water, when allowed to cool to lukewarm, then strained and used as an enema, or injected, about an ounce at a time, is a highly recommended remedy for painful and bleeding internal hemorrhoids, said to bring marvelous relief and speedy healing. For more extended treatment of hemorrhoids, Witch-Hazel Suppositories are probably better than infusion injection. Mix 1 part dried witch-hazel leaves powdered fine with 2 parts cocoa butter and shape into little suppositories about the size of the first joint of your little finger. Keep these suppositories in a cool place, and insert one after each bowel movement. I don't guarantee results, but I have known of several severe cases where these suppositories really helped in this condition.

The Indians poured hot water over fresh witch-hazel leaves, then used them as poultices for sprains, bruises, and swellings, applying the wilted leaves as hot as the patient could comfortably stand them. This was said not only to aid in eventual cure, but also to relieve immediate pain.

Although no outstanding medicinal properties have been detected in witch-hazel, that does not mean that none exists, for, despite its long use in medicine, this plant has been only partially explored. It contains several little-known or unknown substances, and any one of these might prove to be an outstanding healing agent. It has never, to my knowledge, been tested for its antibiotic activity, and it should be. I would not be at all surprised if some day medical science announced that witch-hazel had proved to be a more efficacious healer than it had formerly been thought to be. Meanwhile, I will continue to use witch-hazel preparations on empirical grounds. I feel that they help, and my feelings are pretty important when it is my pain that is being relieved and my complaints that are being cured.

5. Comforting Composites:
BONESET, COLTSFOOT, AND YARROW

THIS PLANT is also called "thoroughwort," "Indian sage," and "vegetable antimony" in some parts of its very extensive range. Probably no other wild American herb has been as widely and continuously used in home remedies as boneset. Our knowledge of the virtues of the plant came from the Indians, and some of its many common names are translations of the original Indian terms. Thousands of country people still gather and use this herb regularly and would consider a home without a good supply of dried boneset very poorly prepared for possible family illnesses. In searching the old herbals for lore on home remedies I find boneset recommended for fevers, colds, rheumatism, catarrh, dropsy, bilious fevers, dengue fever, general debility, dyspepsia, influenza, pneumonia, troubles arising from intemperance, lake fever (an old term for typhoid), and many other illnesses too numerous to mention. No wonder it has long been a valued home remedy. With boneset in the house, other medicines would hardly seem necessary. The value of boneset in at least some of these conditions has been officially recognized, and the herb and some of its preparations have been listed in the U.S. *Pharmacopeia* and the U.S. *Dispensatory*.

One reason why boneset has been so popular in home remedies is its wide availability. It grows in swamps, bogs, low places, pond shores, and stream sides, from Canada to Florida and west to Texas and Nebraska. The single stout stem reaches a height of three to four feet, and the plant is instantly recognizable by its peculiar leaves,

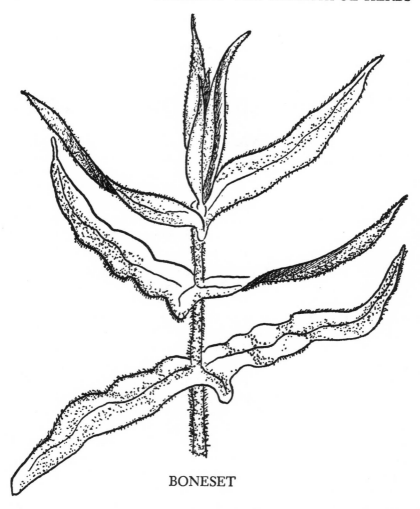

BONESET

which are opposite, slender and pointed, joined together around the stem at their bases and giving the effect of one long leaf, pointed at both ends and pierced at the center by the stem. The leaves are hairy underneath and dark green above, and the vein design gives the upper surface of the leaves a mosaic effect. The single stem branches near the top in late summer, and each branch produces a large head of white flowers.

Gather your supply of boneset just before the plants start to flower, and dry the herb in the shade. As with most other plants mentioned in this book, I merely spread the boneset plants on clean paper in my warm, airy attic, and they always have dried perfectly in one week. Crumble the plant coarsely, remove all large stems, store the dried herb in airtight jars, and it will keep until boneset is ready to harvest next year. All herbs lose virtue by long storage, so renew your supply every year.

My Pennsylvania Dutch neighbors make only one medicine of boneset, but they use it in treating many minor complaints and swear by its efficacy. They also sometimes swear *at* its taste, for it is bitter and astringent. Pour 1 pint of boiling water over 1 heaping tablespoonful of the herb, let it infuse for 30 minutes, then strain. For feverish colds and influenza the patient is kept in bed and given one wineglassful of the tea, as hot as he can drink it, every half-hour until four doses are taken. This usually induces sweating, drives down the fever, and brings great relief to the aches and pains accompanying such conditions. They maintain that this treatment will often break up and dissipate an incipient cold. Maybe it does. How can you prove that a cold has been prevented?

For general debility, dyspepsia, loss of appetite, or other conditions in which a tonic seems to be indicated, they take the infusion cold, in wineglass doses, about 30 minutes before each meal. This is continued for as much as a week, or as long as the condition persists. It seems that boneset is one of the many natural "bitter tonics" so widely distributed among the wild herbs.

COLTSFOOT OR COUGHWORT
(*Tussilago Farfara*)

The botanical name of this plant, *Tussilago*, means "cough dispeller," and it is one of the finest herbal cough medicines. In former days this remedy became so widely known and was so highly esteemed that the plant came to symbolize all herbal medicine. When most of the populace was illiterate, the apothecaries of France painted a coltsfoot leaf on the door, so those who could not read would know that herbal medicines were sold there. Coltsfoot has been called "nature's best herb for the lungs and her most eminent thoracic." Dioscorides, Galen, Pliny, and other ancient physicians praised its healing powers, and it is still considered one of the safest and most

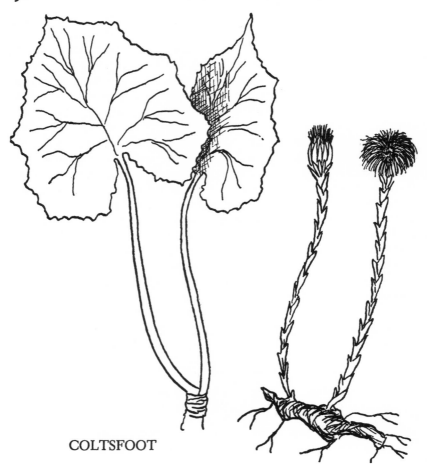

COLTSFOOT

efficacious ways of treating a cough. I sometimes wonder if the popularity of coltsfoot as a cough remedy is not as much due to its flavor
as to its efficacy, for whether taken as cough drops, syrup, or tea, it is
one of the most palatable of all cough remedies. There is never any
difficulty in getting either children or adults to take this remedy
when it is needed, for after acquiring a taste for coltsfoot flavor one
seems to crave it, and I often suck on a coltsfoot cough drop purely
for pleasure.

Botanically the plant is an oddity. It is one of the first flowers to appear in the spring, rivaling the dandelion and the skunk cabbage in this respect. It has perennial spreading white roots, and from these, often in late February, appear little flower stalks resembling tiny asparagus shoots. There are some very small, scale-like clasping leaves on this little seedstalk that have no resemblance to the true leaves, which appear later. When the flower opens, the coltsfoot ceases to resemble undersized asparagus and starts to mimic the dandelion, to which it is actually related. The flower is somewhat similar to the dandelion in color, form, and size, and even turns into the same kind of fuzzball or blowball when it seeds. After the flowers are gone, the leaves tardily appear, springing from separate buds on the perennial root. These leaves are large, two to six inches across, and the plant is called coltsfoot because the outline of the leaves is thought to resemble the track of a young horse. They are roughly rounded and heart-shaped with wavy or sinuate edges, and the margins are toothed. The veins are prominent, and on the under side of the leaf they are covered with fine, cobwebby hairs.

The habit of producing its leaves and flowers at different times caused ancient botanists to think these were two separate plants, and they classed the coltsfoot flower as a leafless plant. This seems inexcusably poor observation, for the leaves often appear before the last of the old fluff-heads from the flowers have disintegrated. The leaves are the part most often used in herbal remedies, and they should be gathered in June or July. Cough drops and cough syrup are better made from the fresh leaves, while Coltsfoot Tea is made from the dried leaves.

To make your own Coltsfoot Cough Drops, cover 1 ounce of fresh coltsfoot leaves with a pint of water and boil down until there is only 1 cupful of liquid left. Strain, and to the liquid add 2 cups of sugar and boil until a drop of this syrup will form a hard ball when dropped into cold water, or until it reaches 250° on your candy thermometer. Pour onto a buttered cookie sheet and score it into cough-drop sizes before it becomes completely hard. When it has cooled and hardened, break apart and roll the drops in slippery-elm powder so they won't be sticky. To make Coltsfoot Cough Syrup, proceed exactly as in making cough drops except that after the sugar is added the syrup is merely brought to a boil, then bottled. An even more efficacious cough syrup can be made by substituting wild-thyme honey for the sugar, but the strong taste of the thyme honey does mask part of the good flavor of the coltsfoot. Either kind of cough syrup can be taken in tablespoon doses as needed, for they contain no drastic drugs or dangerous ingredients.

The leaves can be dried by simply spreading them on clean papers in a warm room until they are dry enough to crumble. To make Coltsfoot Tea use a tablespoonful of the dried leaves to a cupful of boiling water. Allow it to infuse for 5 minutes, then strain and sweeten to taste with honey. This tea is reputed to be an excellent remedy for coughs, colds, and asthma, but I enjoy the taste of Coltsfoot Tea so well that I frequently drink it for pure pleasure.

Another way to use dried coltsfoot leaves is to smoke them like tobacco, for stubborn coughs, asthma, or bronchitis. We have all heard stories about how frightened Europeans were when they first saw returning New World explorers smoking tobacco, but these stories must be apocryphal, for Europeans had been familiar with smoking coltsfoot and other herbs for medicinal reasons for ages before tobacco was introduced there. They had not, however, developed pipes, cigarettes, or cigars, which were American Indian inventions, but inhaled the smoke from burning herbs in a more primitive manner.

Pliny, the great Greco-Roman naturalist of the 1st century, gives directions for smoking coltsfoot that sound like a religious rite, indicating that this practice was well developed by his time. He directed that one build a tiny fire of cypress charcoal, drop dried and crumbled coltsfoot leaves on it, and inhale the smoke through a hollow reed, taking a sip of wine between puffs. This was recommended for every chest ailment from "humours and distillations on the lungs" to such minor complaints as wheezes and stitches in the side. He does not say how large the sips of wine should be, nor how long the process should be continued. My own experiments with this method indicate that when the hollow reed looks double, it is time to slow down, and when it begins to resemble a set of panpipes, it is time to quit.

The smoking of coltsfoot has enjoyed uninterrupted popularity from before Pliny's time down to the present day. One can still buy British Herb Tobacco in which the chief ingredient is coltsfoot. This so-called tobacco also contains eyebright, buckbean, betony, rosemary, thyme, and lavender, but no real tobacco at all. It is mild and fragrant when smoked in a pipe, but it doesn't satisfy the craving for tobacco, and is taken to cure coughs and wheezes, not as a substitute for the "filthy weed."

This British product contains too many domestic herbs for my wild taste, so I set about devising a herbal smoking mixture made entirely of wild plants I can gather in my own neighborhood. The blend I finally devised is better, I believe, than the old-country product, both in flavor and in medicinal efficacy. The herbs I use are all dried and coarsely crumbled, with the stems and leaf veins picked out. I use 8 ounces of coltsfoot, 2 ounces each of mullein, bearberry, and deer-tongue leaves, and 1 ounce each of wild thyme, peppermint, dried rose petals, and fine-cut sassafras-root bark. When smoked in a pipe it is exceedingly fragrant and really seems to relieve a cough and stop wheezes. When it is about half used, I add a half-pound of aromatic pipe tobacco, which makes a more satisfying if less healthful smoke that still perfumes a room like burning incense. It is my hope that all these healing herbs will undo the damage being wrought by tobacco and allow me to enjoy this ancient American Indian herb, which I love altogether too well, with a clear conscience.

YARROW, MILFOIL, OR WOUNDWORT
(Achillea Millefolium)

Here is a pretty little immigrant that has become so common in pastures, meadows, and wastelands that we tend to overlook it altogether or dismiss it as a weed. We make little or no use of it, and yet, back in its Old World native lands it has been used to stanch the blood of battle wounds, to cast spells, to conjure up the devil, to make love charms, to make herbal medicines said to cure a host of ills, to brew a highly intoxicating beer, and, as a shampoo, to prevent baldness. Since it is reputed to have so many abilities, surely we can find a few jobs for this handsome little herb to do.

Yarrow is not a native of America; it was probably brought here by some herbalist among the early settlers for its medicinal uses. It quickly escaped and made itself thoroughly at home in this country, growing in the grass of almost every roadside. It stands ten to twenty inches tall, with leaves three to four inches long and about one inch across, clasping the angular stem with their bases. These leaves are twice-pinnate, that is, they are shaped like a feather and each of the little lateral segments is also formed like a tiny feather, giving this foliage a very feathery appearance indeed. Yarrow blossoms from June until October. The individual flowers are very small, but they tend to cluster at the top of the plant in large flat heads, white or pale rose in color. For making herbal medicines, yarrow should be gathered while in bloom and dried in a warm room.

Like all plants that have entered deeply into herbal medicine and folklore, yarrow is known by a number of different names. Its most ancient use was as a vulnerary, a first-aid treatment of wounds received in battle, and the botanical name *Achillea* refers to a legend that Achilles first revealed the healing power of this herb and used it to treat soldiers wounded in the siege of Troy. Obviously, it did not heal the wound made by an arrow shot by Paris that struck Achilles on the heel. This early use of yarrow is reflected in such folk names as "soldier's woundwort," "knight's milfoil," "*herbe militaris*," "bloodwort," "stanchweed," and "sanguinary." Even the common name "carpenter's weed" refers to its use in treating the cuts and scratches that carpenters were apt to suffer from their many sharp tools.

It is the doubly divided lacy leaves that give the species name, *Millefolium*, which means "thousand-leaves." Such names as "milfoil," "thousand seal," and "thousand weed" also come from this fine-divided foliage. Because yarrow was used in magic spells and divinations, it was also called "devil's nettle" or "devil's plaything." Finally, its pungent taste gave it the name "old man's pepper," and its use in brewing caused it to be called "field hops."

This many-named plant was listed in the old herbals as a vulnerary, styptic, diaphoretic, astringent, tonic, and aromatic, besides its use in magic, charms, and spells. I am sorry that I am not familiar enough with the use of yarrow in conjuring up the devil to explain how it is done. I never need such charms or spells to summon the devil. All it takes is a few idle thoughts and a moment of inattention, and the old boy is right at my elbow suggesting something we can do or something we can leave undone. What I need are some of the many herbs that are reputed to keep that visitor away.

I can tell you how to make one of the many love charms that have been made with yarrow. This one is not nearly as messy as the charm made with wormwood. You merely sew an ounce of the herb

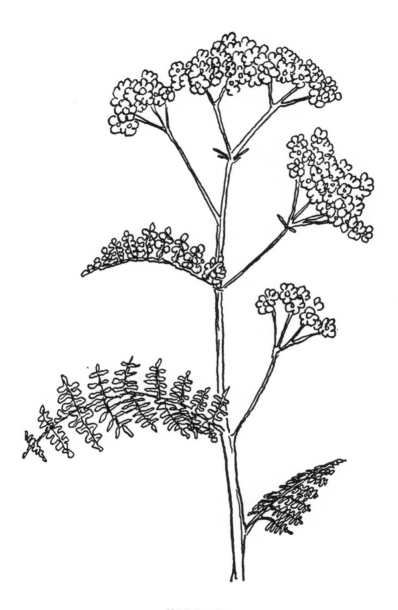

YARROW

into a little square of flannel and place it under your pillow. Before going to bed, recite the following formula in a singsong intonation:

"Thou pretty herb of Venus' tree,
  Thy true name is yarrow
Now who my bosom friend must be,
  Pray tell thou me tomorrow."

If all has been properly done, just before you awaken the next morning you will see your future husband or wife in a vision. Presumably this only works with single boys and girls, though with divorce becoming so common, I don't see why it should be entirely limited to them.

The great Swedish botanist, Linnaeus, recommended the bruised raw fresh herb as an excellent vulnerary and styptic, to be applied to fresh wounds to stop the bleeding and heal the cut. This might also relieve some of the pain, for yarrow seems to have some powers as a local anesthetic, as the fresh leaves are sometimes chewed—despite their pungency and bitter astringency—to relieve toothache. Linnaeus is also the authority for the statement that beer brewed with yarrow is much more intoxicating than that made when hops are used.

The most commonly used home remedy of yarrow is the now-familiar infusion made by pouring 1 pint of boiling water over 1 ounce of the dried herb. You can even use that ounce of yarrow you sewed up in the square of flannel, as dreaming over it doesn't appreciably reduce its strength. This infusion is given hot, in wine-glassful doses, and to each dose is added 1 teaspoonful of honey and 3 drops of Tabasco sauce. If this hot infusion is sipped when the patient is in bed and heavily covered, it is supposed to be an excellent treatment for severe colds, fevers, and the early stages of measles. It opens the pores and causes copious sweating, and in measles it is said to help bring out the spots and shorten the illness. It is also said to "purify the blood" and "flush the kidneys," and presumably anyone who has such low resistance that his body develops any kind of illness needs these things done.

Finally, this same infusion, unsweetened and unpeppered, is said to prevent baldness if the head be washed regularly with it. I mention in the chapter on cleavers that when women learn of that herb's value in reducing diets, I expect to see a million overweight women out combing the countryside for cleavers. Now, I expect these million women will meet a million men with thinning hair, out harvesting the abundant crop of yarrow. The prospects for middle-aged romances are incalculable. Yarrow is a benign herb with some very interesting possibilities.

6. Wild Lettuce:

A VEGETABLE TRANQUILIZER

(*Lactuca canadensis* and *L. scariola*)

THERE are two kinds of wild lettuce common over nearly all of North America, the native wild lettuce, *Lactuca canadensis*, commonly called tall lettuce, or horseweed, and the prickly lettuce, *L. scariola*, also called compass plant, which originally came from Europe, but is now found as an extremely common and bothersome weed in cultivated ground all over the United States. Both species seem to have trouble deciding whether to be annuals or biennials, sometimes flowering and seeding the first year and sometimes delaying this operation until the second year.

The native *tall lettuce*, or *horseweed*, *L. canadensis*, is found from Nova Scotia to British Columbia, south to Georgia and Louisiana, and west at least as far as New Mexico. It thrives in low, damp places, in permanent hay meadows, and along fencerows, and seldom becomes a bad weed. The prefix "horse," when applied to plants, usually means large, coarse, and rank-growing, as horseradish, horse chestnut, horsemint, etc. Horseweed grows from four to nine feet tall, but in this case the name is doubly apt, for horses love the flavor of lettuce and will eat this weed avidly. The lower leaves are variable in shape, deeply cut like an oversized dandelion leaf, and from five to twelve inches long. The stem leaves clasp the stem with their bases, are variously cut and toothed, bright green on top and whitish underneath. The upper leaves on the seed stalk are often lance-shaped with entire margins that are neither toothed nor lobed. The flower stalk branches near the summit and produces numerous urn-shaped flower heads about a half-inch tall, with yellow flowers having numerous strap-shaped petals.

The introduced weed, prickly lettuce, *L. scariola*, is now far more common and abundant than our native wild tall lettuce. Most botanists believe that it is the original ancestor of all our many varieties of garden lettuce, but it is only when the wild plant is very young that one is likely to notice the family resemblance. Prickly lettuce is also sometimes called horseweed and deserves the name, for it grows from two to seven feet tall and when young and tender it is eagerly eaten by horses. When the bright yellow-green leaves first appear in the spring, the plant closely resembles young leaf lettuce from the garden, in both taste and appearance, but it sends up a seedstalk that may be several feet high by mid-May, and by August it sometimes towers over a tall man. The stem leaves are pinnate, or deeply cut, with sharp-toothed margins, almost bristle-tipped. The lower leaves are six to eight inches long, with those toward the top of the stalk smaller. The bases of these leaves have earlike, backward projections that clasp the stalk. A peculiar feature of these leaves is that they twist and turn during the day, keeping one edge toward the sun, and for this reason the prickly lettuce is sometimes called the compass plant. The lower part of the stem and the midribs of the leaves are covered with weak prickles. It frequents fields, waste places, and roadsides, and is often a troublesome weed.

These two species have similar medical properties, or lack of them, and both are equally edible, so from here on we can treat them alike. When one of the tall seedstalks is broken or cut, a thick, white, milky juice exudes, which soon coagulates and stiffens into a rubber-like consistency. This gum turns a reddish-brown on long exposure to the air. Formerly great quantities of this gum were gathered and sold to the drug trade, it being considered only slightly less valuable than opium. It looks like opium, smells like opium, and even tastes a bit like raw opium, but modern medical science says that it has few, if any, of the physiological effects of opium, and is, at best, only a very weak sedative. It was formerly used as a substitute for opium in treating nervous illnesses, for insomnia, for allaying the pain of rheumatism and colic, to relieve coughing, and to treat diarrhea. I cautiously experimented with this gum, but could notice no effects whatever from the small doses I took. Maybe I didn't use the right recipe. One old book of home remedies says to dissolve three lumps of this gum, each the size of a pea, in a quart of brandy, and to give this tincture *in 2- to 4-ounce doses* for sleeplessness. Well! A few doses of brandy that size would do something—whether it contained wild lettuce gum or not. Even if it didn't put the patient to sleep, it would probably make him perfectly happy to stay awake.

As usual, I would rather eat my wild herbs as food than take them as medicine. When the first leaves of either kind of wild lettuce are only a few inches high, they make splendid salads, especially when mixed with other salad materials. At this stage they taste like young leaf lettuce from the garden, only more so. Unfortunately, wild lettuce stays in this eminently edible condition only a week or so. As the season advances, it develops a bitter flavor that gradually becomes stronger, until by the time the seedstalk appears it is totally inedible. Good as wild lettuce is in salads, it is even better when cooked, being one of the most delicious of all potherbs. When gathered very young it is so tender that it requires very little cooking, so that it can be served with its vitamins and minerals still intact.

The easiest way to cook wild lettuce is to gather the leaves, wash them, and place them in a covered saucepan. The water that clings to the leaves will furnish all the cooking water necessary. Bring them to a boil; then cook, covered, for only 2 minutes. Season with butter and salt, and serve. An even better way is to cook 2 slices of bacon, chopped fine, until it is crisp, then add as many lettuce leaves as the pan will hold, cover and shake them around until they are all evenly coated with the bacon fat, then cook only until they are hot through. This wild lettuce is not so much cooked as merely wilted. Add a little vinegar and some raw onion, chopped fine, and serve hot.

This wild lettuce shrinks to only a fraction of its former bulk when cooked, and one can thus eat much more of it as a cooked green than as a salad. I never noticed any physiological or psychological effects from eating wild lettuce salads, but when I ate a large helping of the cooked greens I became aware of a sort of languid drowsiness and feeling of well-being, as though I didn't have a care in the world. This happened several times after eating fairly large amounts of this vegetable, and I don't think it was just my imagination. The only trouble with this wild tranquilizer is that it is available such a short time of the year. To remedy this I developed a method of freezing these greens. I simply fill a wire strainer or colander with freshly picked wild lettuce leaves, dip it in boiling water for one minute, then quickly cool the vastly shrunken greens under the cold water faucet, pack them into freezer containers or plastic bags, and put them in the freezer. Now, whenever I feel nervous or irritable, I merely lunch or dine on wild lettuce greens and then bask in a feeling of complete relaxation.

7. Medicine and Magic from Wormwood

(*Artemisia Absinthium*)

WORMWOOD has been surrounded by an aura of superstition and awe since ancient times. From early biblical days it has been used in medicine and magic, as a bitter flavoring herb and to mingle with wine to make it more intoxicating. In ancient Greece this herb was sacred to Artemis, the nature goddess, and from her, some people think, the genus gets its botanical name. Artemis was both a goddess of healing and a purveyor of death, and wormwood, like the opium poppy, is a blessing when properly used and a curse when misused. When combined with alcohol in liqueurs, as in absinthe, it has a deleterious effect when taken in excess. In the United States, it is illegal to manufacture or import absinthe. When properly used, wormwood is a stimulating bitter tonic that can be a great blessing to those in a debilitated condition who are suffering from poor appetite and enfeebled digestion.

Wormwood is one of the bitterest of all herbs, but it is a noble bitter. This species is not native to America, but has been widely naturalized and is now found growing wild through the northeastern states from the Atlantic Coast to the Great Plains. It seems to prefer the vicinity of man and is most common along roadsides and near dwellings, seldom being found in remote areas. It has a perennial root, and from it each spring rises the feathery, greenish-white foliage. The basal leaves, about three inches long and half that broad, are segmented, the segments segmented, and these segments further seg-

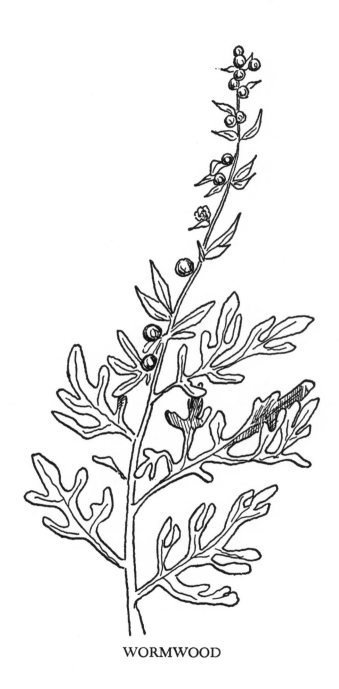

WORMWOOD

mented, making a very lacy, thrice-pinnate leaf that is quite attractive. The sparse flower stalk rises about two feet, bearing a few small leaves of three segments and some even smaller ones of only one linear segment each. The whole plant has a grayish look, being covered with very fine silky hairs. The small composite flowers, almost globular, are greenish-yellow in color and hang downward from the branched flower stalk.

The leaves and flowers of wormwood are used together in the herbal remedies. Collect the whole herb in July or August and hang it in a warm room until dry. When thoroughly dry, crumble and rub through a coarse sieve to remove the larger stems. Pack the crumbled herb loosely in a fruit jar. Set the open jar in a slow oven for about half an hour so it will be warmed through, then seal with a domed lid. This will keep the dry herb from reabsorbing moisture during damp weather.

Wormwood has always had a high place in magic, and the following love charm is from medieval England. On Saint Luke's Eve, October 18, mix together a thimbleful each of wormwood, dried marigold flowers, dried marjoram, and dried thyme, all crumbled fine. Add half a cup of water, and simmer over low heat for 7 minutes, then strain. To the liquid add a thimbleful of virgin honey and a thimbleful of vinegar, mix well, and anoint yourself all over with the resultant goo. Then repeat three times:

> "Saint Luke, Saint Luke, be kind to me,
> In dreams let me my true love see."

Get into bed and that night you will dream of the one you will marry.

I must admit that I haven't tried this charm. Not only have I been thoroughly and completely married for lo these many years, but the whole process sounds a bit messy. Isn't virgin honey sticky? For that matter, what is virgin honey? All honey is made by worker bees, and they are all undeveloped females, presumably living and dying virgins. Still there are naturalists who go into ecstacies over the marvelous way of life the bees have. I could think of some improvements. Maybe Saint Luke and wormwood should do something for the producers of virgin honey.

Wormwood can also be combined with honey to make a stimulating cordial for internal use. Put 2 ounces of crumbled wormwood in a quart jar and pour 1 pint of good brandy over it. Let it macerate for 48 hours (shake the jar occasionally), then strain and to the liquid add a half-cupful of honey and enough green food coloring to give it a pretty tint. This is not absinthe, but a wormwood cordial, and it can be given in half-ounce doses for faintness or near-swooning. It can also be served in liqueur glasses as a luxurious finish to a fine dinner, and you needn't tell your guests that it will also prevent after-eating distress.

Besides its use in absinthe and cordial, wormwood has also been used in making wine and beer. Before brewers finally settled on hops as the proper bitter herb to use in beer, they experimented with many others, among them wormwood, which not only gave beer the coveted bitter flavor but also increased its intoxicating power. Why hops finally won out over wormwood in the brewing industry is anybody's guess, for, from all reports, a glass of wormwood beer had considerably more kick than one brewed with hops.

One 18th-century herbalist writes that Germans made wormwood wine by "working" the herb with the wine expressed from grapes ("working" means fermenting, in wine making). He says "it is strong and an excellent wine, not unpleasant, yet of such efficacy to give an appetite that the Germans drink a glass with every other mouthful, and that way eat for hours together, without sickness or indigestion." It sounds absolutely gruesome, and his account is obviously grossly exaggerated, if not entirely untrue. That much wine would be deadly, no matter what herbs were mixed with it, and so much wormwood would probably be fatal even if one could survive that much food. You'd better not try it.

Probably the best way to take wormwood is in that almost standard herb infusion made by pouring 1 pint of boiling water over 1 ounce of the herb. In this case allow the herb to infuse overnight, and next day decant off the clear liquid. Keep it in the refrigerator and take it cold, a wineglassful at a dose, a half-hour before dinner. This is the now-familiar bitter tonic, which, by increasing the flow of gastric juices, is supposed to rouse a languid appetite and stimulate digestion. In addition, some herbalists say that this infusion will give a feeling of mental alertness and general well-being. I could discern no stimulating effect from wineglassful doses. A cup of coffee gives me more lift. However, wormwood does contain some drugs that are stimulants to the central nervous system, and if you notice that it

gives you a good feeling, don't pursue it, for an overdose of wormwood can definitely be harmful.

The old herbalists sing the praises of this wormwood infusion with
no uncertain sound. One says it will "relieve melancholia" and cure
"the hypochondriacal disorders of studious, sedentary men." Another
says that if this infusion is taken for a week, one "will have no sickness after meals, will feel none of that fulness so frequent from indigestion, and wind will be no more troublesome." Truly a noble
herb, this wormwood.

8. Elecampane, Horseheal, or Elf Dock

(*Inula Helenium*)

> Let no day pass without eating some of the roots of ele-
> campane condited [pickled, preserved], to help digestion,
> to expel melancholy and sorrow and to cause mirth.
>
> —PLINY

THE QUOTATION above shows that the use of elecampane in
herbal medicine goes back many centuries. Unlike many medicines of antiquity, this one has retained the respect of modern doctors
and is still listed in most pharmacopoeias. It has the possibility of
burgeoning into one of the modern, scientific wonder drugs, if those
searching for antibiotics among higher plants ever get around to
testing this promising plant. I know that elecampane root makes an
interesting confection, with a fascinating bitter-sweet-aromatic flavor
that one comes to crave.

Elecampane came to America as a healer, being introduced into
gardens for use in home remedies. It found a congenial climate here
and rapidly went native, now being found wild throughout the Eastern and Central States. This relative of the lowly daisy is a strikingly
handsome plant with a stout, deeply furrowed stem that reaches a
height of four to five feet, branched near its summit. The basal leaves
are often more than a foot long and four inches wide, ovate-pointed
in shape, with serrated margins, and so downy they feel like velvet.
The leaves on the stem are proportionately shorter and broader, with

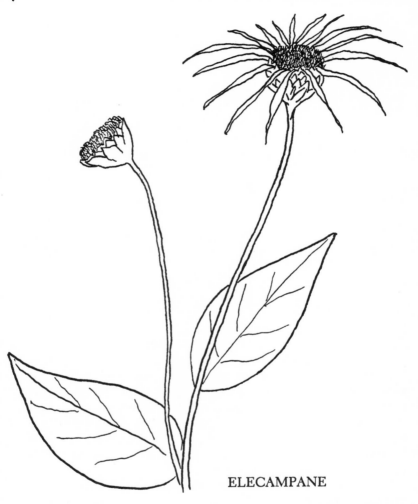

ELECAMPANE

stem-clasping bases. The blossoms appear in July and August, each
one three to four inches across, bright-yellow, and resembling a
double sunflower. The perennial rootstock is top-shaped or spindle-
shaped, often branching, succulent, brown in color, and slightly
aromatic in odor. Look for this plant in damp, rocky meadows or
pastures, often growing where it is partly shaded.

The ancient Greeks and Romans valued elecampane, not only as an efficacious medicine, but also as a culinary herb and condiment. Even the poets were acquainted with it, and Horace, in one of his poems, mentions a delicate sauce made of it and also says that Romans who had eaten, not wisely but too well, pined for elecampane to relieve their distress. Among the common people of Rome there was a Latin couplet-aphorism that went, "Enula campana / reddit praecordia sana," which would translate, "Elecampane will lift your spirits." The herb was described and its medicinal virtues were extolled by such respected ancient doctors as Pliny and Dioscorides. Pliny even asserts that "the root, being chewed fasting doth fasten loose teeth," while Galen, who is, after Hippocrates, the most celebrated physician of antiquity, says, according to the quaint English translation before me, "It is good for passions of the hucklebone."

I know I could easily learn what part of the anatomy was meant by the term "hucklebone," but I refuse to do so. I prefer that my hucklebone be without precise location or definition, so that it can be assigned to any place or function my imagination dictates. It is good to know that I can allay its passions by eating a piece of candied elecampane. At the same time—I have Pliny's word for it—this simple confection will expel melancholy and sorrow and cause mirth. What more could you want? Besides, I like the stuff.

The substance most abundantly contained in elecampane root is *inulin*, a sort of invert starch that has often been recommended as a replacement for ordinary starch in the diets of diabetics. It also contains a volatile oil and several named crystallizable substances; it is to these minor constituents that its drug action is thought to be due. The listed medicinal actions are: diuretic, tonic, diaphoretic, expectorant, alterative, antiseptic, astringent, and gently stimulant. English herbalists have long used elecampane in treating coughs, consumption, and chronic diseases of the lungs. It is still a favorite home remedy for bronchitis and asthma, and is said to relieve difficult breathing and to expel phlegm by assisting expectoration.

An English herbalist of the 17th century, writing about elecampane, tells us, "It is good for shortness of the breathe and an old cough, and for such as cannot breathe unless they hold their neckes upright." Another herbalist of the same century says, "The fresh roots of Elecampane preserved with sugar are very effectual to warm a cold, windy stomach and stitches in the side, caused by spleen and to relieve cough, shortness of the breath and wheezing in the lungs."

The name *"horseheal"* was given to this plant in England, where it is still sometimes used by veterinarians to treat pulmonary complaints of horses. Modern researchers may prove that all these uses of elecampane in pulmonary diseases were justified. From several sources, including the *U.S. Dispensatory*, we learn that as far back as 1885, a Dr. Korab, who was experimenting wth elecampane, demonstrated that the active bitter principle of the plant, called *helenin*, was a powerful antiseptic and bactericide, a solution of as little as 1 part in 10,000 immediately killing ordinary bacterial organisms, and Dr. Korab remarked that it was particularly destructive to the tubercle bacillus.

This account was to me an exciting find, indicating that as far back as 1885 a researcher was stumbling around on the very threshold of the science of antibiotics, nearly a half-century before Dr. Fleming discovered penicillin and ushered in some of the most potent healers of modern medicine. The search for medicinally useful antibiotics among the higher plants is still in its infancy, although some promising finds have already been made. (See page 212.) It seems to me that sufficient evidence exists, indicating that elecampane probably contains some powerful antibiotic substance, to warrant a thorough exploration of this interesting herb.

Such sophisticated research is for organizations with huge budgets and large facilities. My primary interest has been to learn how ordinary people can gather, prepare, and use this unusual herb, for elecampane, because it contains no drastic or dangerous drugs, is singularly adapted to home use. The large plant is very conspicuous when in flower, so this is the time to select your future foraging grounds. Delay the actual digging until late autumn, however. Discard or replace all old, woody roots, and scrub those you select with a stiff brush and cold water. Cut each root crosswise into 2-inch lengths, then slice each piece lengthwise into 4 to 8 segments. To 2 cups of prepared pieces add 2 cups of water and 2 cups of sugar. Bring to a boil, then reduce the heat and barely simmer until the elecampane is tender.

This gives you two products, Candied Elecampane, and Elecampane Syrup. Drain the elecampane and bottle the syrup. This syrup is reputed to be an excellent cough remedy, either used by itself or combined with various other herbal medicines. After draining thoroughly, allow the Candied Elecampane to dry on waxed paper for two days, then roll in granulated sugar, let dry another day, and store in tight jars. This Candied Elecampane can be nibbled for coughs and breathing difficulties, or solely for its good taste—the reason I eat it—or it can be made into other attractive products.

In studying elecampane, I read that this herb has been used in France and Switzerland to flavor gins, absinthe, and cordials, so I started intensive experiments in this field, a task that involved several of my drinking friends giving their time and attention to this project. Because of their willing sacrifices, you can now enjoy the recipe that they agreed made the very best Elecampane Liqueur of them all.

You will need 1 quart of fresh red currants, 1 quart of good brandy, and 2 cups of Candied Elecampane Roots. Crush the currants, a layer at a time, until they are thoroughly mashed. Add a half-cup of water and simmer for 10 minutes, then strain out the juice through a jelly bag. This will give you about 1 pint of bright-red juice. To this, add 2 cups of sugar while the juice is still hot, and stir until the sugar is thoroughly dissolved, then when cool, add the quart of brandy. Find 2 quart bottles with mouths wide enough so that you can get the elecampane into them and put a cup of Candied Elecampane into each. Pour the mixed brandy and currant juice over the elecampane, seal the bottles, store them in a dark place, and don't touch them for a month. The longer the elecampane is left in, the stronger the flavor it imparts, and even when the liqueur is finished, the brandy-flavored pieces of Candied Elecampane make an exotic nibble. This is the elecampane preparation that dispels melancholy and provokes mirth.

Early in the 19th century, Elecampane Candy was a favorite sweet of English schoolboys, and some thought that the prowess of English boys on the athletic field could be attributed partly to their consumption of elecampane, for this herb is supposed to strengthen the wind, improve endurance, and prevent stitches in the side of those who play hard. Dr. Fernie, writing early in this century, said, "Some fifty years ago, the candy was sold commonly in London as flat, round cakes, being composed largely of sugar and colored with cochineal. A piece was eaten each night and morning for asthmatical complaints."

I determined to re-create this interesting ancient remedy, and the candy I finally produced, while surely not identical with the old product, is, I believe, as delicious as any ever produced by an English confectioner. To make Elecampane Candy, put a half-teaspoon of baking soda and 1 cup of sugar into a saucepan, mix thoroughly, then add a half-cup of light cream. Bring to a boil over medium high heat and cook, stirring occasionally, until it reaches the soft-ball stage, or shows exactly 234° on your candy thermometer. Remove from heat, stir in 1 level tablespoon of butter, then stir in 1 cupful of Candied Elecampane Root, chopped fine. Beat until thick—2 or 3 minutes—then drop by the teaspoonful on waxed paper. This should make about two dozen little round cakes, and, according to Dr. Fernie, you are limited to two per day. Solely in the interests of science, I experimented, and found that a few more caused me no trouble.

Does this delicious candy really have any value as a medicine? Whether it will cure consumption, bronchitis, asthma, or other pulmonary complaints, I cannot say, for I have never been bothered by any of these diseases and, not being a doctor, I do not prescribe for others. However, I can vouch for some of the other virtues of this wonderful herb. Just the sight of a patch of elecampane blooming by the roadside will lift my spirits and dispel melancholy, and since I have been eating Elecampane Candy regularly, the passions of my hucklebone have been, as far as I can tell, under perfect control.

9. For Courage:

BORAGE, STAR-FLOWER, OR BEEBREAD

(*Borago officinalis*)

IT MAKETH a man merrie and joyfull. Use the floures in sallads to exhilarate and make the minde glad. Used everywhere for the comfort of the heart, for driving away sorrow and increasing the joy of the minde. The leaves and floures of Borage put into wine make men and women glad and merrie and drive away all sadness, dulnesse and melancholie. Syrup made of the floures of Borage comforteth the heart, purgeth melancholie and quieteth the phrenticke and lunaticke person."

Thus one ancient herbalist sings the praise of borage. Another writes, "Hath an excellent spirit to repress the fuliginous vapours of duskie melancholie." While still another says, "Sprigs of Borage are of known virtue to revive the hypochondriac and cheer the hard student." After reading these accounts my first thought was, "What have I been missing?" and I could hardly wait to try this herb. It sounds like the substance the whole world is seeking, the miracle drug for modern ills.

I have seen borage growing unused and unnoticed about dumps, waste places, and old abandoned gardens, but it really can't be called a wild plant in this country. I am partial to wild plants, but in the case of this wonder herb I cheated; I'll admit it. One spring, when I hired a neighbor to disk my orchard, I followed him about and sprinkled borage seed in all the sunny places between the fruit trees. Borage reseeds itself freely, and now, several years after the initial cheat, I have an abundance of "wild" borage growing in my orchard. I use it through the summer to add a cucumber flavor to my salads, to make cooling summer drinks, and to make into confections, jams, jellies, and syrups, so that I can expel the dusky vapors of melancholy the year round.

The best way to learn to recognize this joyful herb is to plant a packet of borage seeds and watch the plants that grow from them. The whole plant is usually about a foot high with large, dark-green, hairy, obovate leaves and beautiful star-shaped blue flowers. Borage is worth raising as an ornamental, and bees prefer these blossoms to all others. Use the leaves as soon as they are large enough, pulling them singly from the plant so the herb can go right on producing another crop of leaves and an abundance of blue flowers.

The reputed medicinal effects of borage are not all due to ancient imaginations. The herb is an excellent source of organic potassium, calcium, and other natural minerals, and it probably rates fairly high in several essential vitamins, although it has not been explored for these latter nutrients. The juice is mucilaginous and soothing to the stomach, adding body as well as flavor to cooling drinks. One modern herbalist recommends pouring a pint of boiling water over 1 ounce of the crushed fresh leaves and taking the infusion cold, in wineglassful doses, but this seems to me to show very little imagination in using borage. This method may work well enough for those who like to take medicine, but I like to imbibe my health with delicious food and drink, and when borage is the medicine, this is easily done.

The simplest and one of the best ways to take borage is merely to nibble the leaves fresh from the garden. Or, the leaves or flowers can be added to a tossed salad. This imparts a pleasant and mild cucumber flavor, but this flavor doesn't linger around as persistently as does that of real cucumbers, making it especially desirable for those who like the taste of cucumber but care little for its aftereffects.

Almost as easy is adding crushed borage leaves to lemonade, limeade, or mixed wine drinks. Vary the amount of borage until you know just how much you and your family like. Even better is to put the leaves through a vegetable juicer and use the greenish, mucilaginous juice in mixing drinks. Lemonade seems twice as cooling when a jigger of borage juice is added to each tumblerful, and don't forget all that exhilaration the ancient herbalists promised. We like this

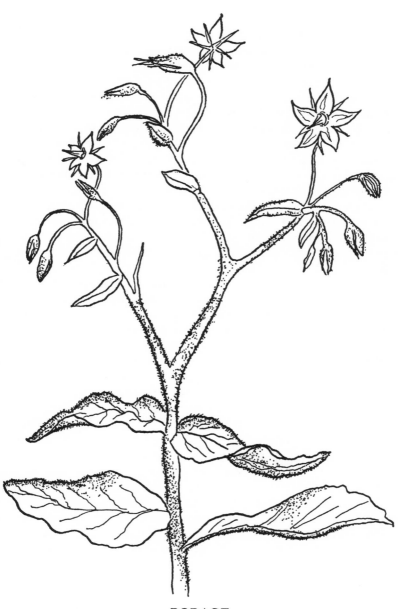

BORAGE

herbal extraction so well that while borage is in full crop I always store a few small jars of juice in the freezer so we can enjoy it with our Christmas wine. I have actually seen borage mixed with wine make both men and women glad and merry, driving away all sadness, dullness, and melancholy, but I suspect the wine content of the drinks had something to do with that. However, the mineral salts in borage can bring a feeling of well-being to anyone whose system is deficient in these nutrients.

To make Borage Syrup, add 2 cups of sugar to 1 cup of borage juice, bring just to a boil, then bottle while still hot. The mucilaginous and demulcent qualities of this syrup will soothe a sore throat, and it has often been recommended for fevers. Certainly it is pleasant to take when mixed with water or lemonade, and the contained mineral salts will no doubt stimulate the kidneys, flushing poisons from the system, while the mineral and vitamin nutrients will help an ill person to regain strength and health.

The candies that I make from borage are Jelly Cubes like those I make from so many wild herbs. Mix together 2 cups sugar and 2 envelopes of unflavored gelatin, then add 1 cup of borage-leaf juice and the juice of 1 lemon. Stir until the sugar is all dissolved and the gelatin well softened. Then add 1 cup boiling water and stir until the gelatin is all dissolved. Rinse a shallow, square mold in cold water, and pour the mixture into it. Allow to cool, then store in the refrigerator until the next day. At that time, mix together 1 cup of powdered sugar and 1 tablespoon of cornstarch. Dip the bottom of the mold into warm water, remove the stiff jelly, and cut it into cubes. Roll each cube in the sugar-starch mixture, and dry on waxed paper. This has a very pleasant lemon-and-borage flavor and a clean taste that never cloys.

You can also candy the star-shaped, blue flowers of borage. Thin the white of 1 egg with 1 tablespoon water and the juice of 1 lemon. Dip the blossoms in this mixture, then roll in granulated sugar. Dry on waxed paper until they will no longer stick together, then put them in a covered glass dish and store in the refrigerator, or in the freezer, if they are to be kept for some time. These are real conversation pieces at parties and as good as they look.

These Candied Borage Blossoms gave me an idea for some Borage Jam. I put 1 cup of borage-leaf juice, made with the vegetable juicer, into an electric blender and added 1 cup of borage blossoms while running the blender at high speed. To this I added the juice of 1 lemon and 2 cups of sugar, then blended them until the sugar was completely dissolved. Then I dissolved 1 package of commercial gelatin in 1 cup water, put it on the heat, brought it to a boil, then boiled hard for 1 minute, stirring constantly until it was melded. This hot pectin mixture was then thoroughly mixed with the borage-sugar mixture and quickly ladled into small jars, covered, and stored in the freezer. I don't use this Borage Jam with meals, but serve small helpings on plain wafers as luxurious party food.

For serving with fish or fowl, I make a Borage-Leaf Jelly, using borage-leaf juice without adding the flowers. To 2 cups borage juice add 3 cups sugar and the juice of 1 lemon, and stir until the sugar is completely dissolved. In a small saucepan, dissolve 1 package commercial pectin in ¾ cup water, then bring to a boil and boil hard for 1 minute, stirring constantly. Thoroughly mix this hot stuff with the borage-sugar mixture, quickly ladle into jelly glasses, cover, and store in the freezer, unless they are to be used in a month or sooner, when the refrigerator will do. This jelly has a distinctive and surprising flavor, and even those who dislike fruit jellies with their meats will welcome borage jelly as a condiment. The idea in making Borage Jam and Borage-Leaf Jelly in this peculiar manner is to avoid cooking the borage, which debases the flavor and destroys some of the valuable nutrients.

All the borage products have been recommended as beneficial to persons weakened by long sickness, and have been given to those afflicted with faintness or swooning. One old-time herbalist even recommends borage for such unlikely things as "the biting of serpents, jaundice, consumption and rheumatism."

I much prefer to think of borage as a pleasant food, rather than as a medicine, and it has not been found to contain any drastic or harmful drugs. The exhilaration that comes from taking borage is due to the natural euphoria of feeding a healthy, well-nourished body with any useful nutrient, and is not due to an intoxicating effect. Here is the lift without the letdown, the kick without the kickback, and one never experiences a hangover from a borage binge.

10. Comfrey, Knitbone, or Healing Herb

(Symphytum officinale)

WHAT'S in a name? Of all the hundreds of herbs that have been used in the healing arts, the herbalists chose this one to bear the name "healing herb," and it seems perfectly able to live up to its name. I consider comfrey nearly an ideal herb for making home remedies for use by amateur herbalists. Since it is nonpoisonous and completely harmless, the dosage is never critical, the remedies are easily compounded, and even professional medical men who have studied the subject will admit that comfrey preparations can be of genuine help in many conditions.

Comfrey is not a native American plant, and therefore we have no American Indian traditions of its use. It was probably brought from England to this country by some herbalist who appreciated its healing powers. It went wild and is now found in moist locations, often in part shade, throughout the northeastern states. It is a close relative of borage, but resembles it very little in appearance. Wild comfrey is seldom more than two feet tall; the lower leaves are large and shaped like the outline of a donkey's ears, and both stem and leaves are covered with fine hairs. The flower racemes are found at the top of the plant, bearing white or purplish bell-shaped flowers along only one side of a stem that curls like a scorpion's tail. Each flower is followed by four seeds in a little cup. Comfrey blooms from May until frost, and one can find ripe seeds, open flowers, and tiny buds on the same raceme. The root is large and black outside, and the inside is white, fleshy, and very mucilaginous.

In the old days it was believed that taking comfrey preparations internally and binding comfrey poultices to the injured parts would greatly hasten the healing of broken bones. The very name, comfrey, is a corruption of the Latin *con firmo*, referring to this belief, and the botanical name, *Symphytum*, is from the Greek *symphyo*, meaning "to unite." The specific name, *officinale*, means it was on the list of official medicinal herbs. Many of its common English names, such as knitbones, knitback, boneheal, and consolida, are also allusions to its use in healing broken bones.

It is stylish for modern herbalists to smile tolerantly at the old notion that herbal medicines could hurry the healing of broken bones, but I refuse to join these moderns in their lofty disdain of this ancient belief. What causes broken bones to heal swiftly in one person and take months to knit back together in another? Could it not be that in the slow cases the elements necessary for the healing process are absent, or present in such small quantities that healing proceeds very slowly? Analysis shows that comfrey is high in calcium, potassium, and phosphorus, along with many other useful trace minerals, and the green leaves are rich in vitamins A and C, and broken bones simply refuse to heal unless many of these nutrients are present.

Applied externally, comfrey poultices help to reduce swelling, and it is often the swelling of the injured flesh in the fracture area that pushes broken bones apart or causes them to heal crookedly. I am not advocating that fractures be treated at home without a doctor's care. Our medical men are far better prepared to deal with such injuries than were their forefathers, and I believe in taking full advantage of modern techniques, equipment, and medication. I merely want to point out that the old belief that certain herbs could aid in treating fractures was not nearly as ridiculous as some modern writers seem to believe.

Both the leaves and the roots of comfrey are used in home remedies, and the virtues listed for them are: demulcent, emollient, mildly astringent, expectorant, and vulnerary. "Vulnerary" is an old herbalist's term that was applied to any plant used to cure battle wounds. Comfrey root contains edible, tasteless mucilage in large amounts, a little tannin, which accounts for its slight astringency, a very little starch and sugar, and from 0.6 to 0.8 percent of a drug named allantoin. A well-known medical journal says, "Allantoin in aqueous solution in strengths of 0.3 percent has a powerful action in strengthening epithelial formations [the lining of hollow internal organs], and is a valuable remedy not only in external ulceration, but also in ulcers of the stomach and duodenum."

The British publication, *Chemist and Druggist*, after the discovery of allantoin and the ascertaining of its uses, had this to say on the subject:

"Allantoin is a fresh instance of the good judgment of our rustics, especially of old times with regard to the virtues of plants. The great Comfrey, or consound, though it was official with us down to the middle of the eighteenth century, never had a very prominent place in professional practice; but our herbalists were loud in its praise and the country culler of simples held it almost infallible as a remedy for both external and internal wounds, bruises and ulcers, for phlegm, for spitting of blood, ruptures, haemorrhoids, etc. For ulcers of the stomach and liver especially, the root (the part used) was regarded as of sovereign virtue. It is precisely for such complaints as these that Allantoin, obtained from the rhizomes of the plant, is now prescribed."

The old herbalists were completely unstinted in their praise of comfrey. One, writing in the middle of the 16th century, says, "The water of Greater Comfrie druncke helpeth such as are bursten, and that have broken the bone of the legge." I would consider one who had "bursten" almost beyond repair, but these old herbalists had unlimited faith in comfrey. For instance, Nicholas Culpepper, a thoroughly unreliable "astrological botanist" of the 17th century, wrote, "The roots being outwardly applied cure fresh wounds immediately...." I find that "immediately" pretty hard to swallow, but when he goes on to say that bruised comfrey roots are "specially good for ruptures and broken bones, so powerful to consolidate and knit together that if they be boiled with dissevered pieces of flesh in a pot, it will join them together again," then my gullibility is badly strained. I simply don't believe I can cook comfrey root with hamburger and lift out a sirloin steak. If modern herbalists are looking for an ancient superstition to debunk, let them jump on that one and I'll join them. However, let it be recorded that this was far from being a general belief in 17th-century England. The reliable herbalists, doctors, and botanists of that time were just as skeptical as we are today, and they loudly and decisively repudiated Culpepper's writings. However, as Barnum said, there's one born every minute, so Culpepper's writings went through edition after edition, and a small cult of astrological herbalists have continued to believe this charlatan's nonsense down to the present day, and his works are still being published.

Although comfrey will not do all that some old herbalists claimed for it, it is still a reliable and efficacious remedy for many complaints, and the medicines from it are easily made and administered in the home. These remedies are better made of the fresh herb than of the dried products. A decoction of the root is made by putting 1 pint of milk in the top of a double boiler, adding 1 ounce of the crushed or ground root, and cooking over boiling water for 30 minutes. Strain and take in wineglassful doses every 2 hours. This is recommended as a gentle remedy for diarrhea, coughs, croup, and bronchitis, and for stomach and duodenal ulcers. With ½ ounce of witch-hazel leaves added to this milk-comfrey mixture before cooking, the remedy, taken internally, is said to be a great help for hemorrhoids.

Several herbals recommend boiling-water infusions of the leaves, but I know a better way to get the medicinal benefits of comfrey leaves. The very first leaves, gathered in March or April, long before the plant blooms, make a fine dish of greens. This has long been known and enjoyed in the British Isles, although one botanical writer of the last century said that comfrey greens "were not, however, valued by persons of refined taste." I'll bet a shilling he tried to eat some comfrey greens that were already too old when cooked. It is only the very first leaves in early spring that are palatable, and even young, newly formed leaves from older plants won't do. Gathered in its prime, comfrey to me is the equal of spinach and better than chard. In Ireland, comfrey is sometimes eaten as a "cure for defective circulation and poverty of blood," but it can also be eaten for pure pleasure if you like greens. These young leaves have much the same kind of mucilaginous, demulcent properties as the roots, and no doubt would aid in the treatment of the same kind of complaints, such as stomach ulcers.

Today it is recognized that a contributing cause of stomach ulcers is the nervous tension and anxiety that comes with responsibility, peculiarly a complaint of the rich, successful, and influential. If I ever become successful enough to have stomach ulcers, or if I have the misfortune to develop stomach ulcers without even becoming successful, I intend to follow my doctor's instructions about medication, but I will change my diet to include considerable amounts of comfrey. In early spring I will gather great quantities of the tender leaves, blanch them by submerging them in boiling water for about

2 minutes, pack them in containers, and freeze them. I will then be able to have boiled comfrey greens at least once a day, and my beverages will be the comfrey-milk decoction described above and the Comfrey Coffee described below. Incidentally, if I recover I will let the doctor take credit for the cure.

That Comfrey Coffee is really made of three different kinds of roots. I went to a weedy hay meadow and dug some large roots of dandelion and chicory, and along a nearby ditch I dug some good-sized roots of comfrey, about equal quantities of each kind. These were scrubbed well, then roasted in the oven until they were dark brown all the way through, crisp and brittle. The roasting was a long, slow job that took more than 4 hours. These browned roots were then broken up and ground in an ordinary coffee grinder, and the brew was made in a percolator exactly as one makes coffee, same measurements and all. I didn't originate this recipe, but read about it long ago in an old book that comes from England. The book said the beverage would "taste practically the same as ordinary coffee." I didn't expect too much of this brew, for I have frequently heard returning travelers commenting on the taste of "ordinary coffee" as it is made in England, but it turned out to be a pretty good hot beverage of the coffee-substitute class, and the comfrey contributes a smoothness that is not even found in real coffee (but it still isn't coffee).

Both the leaves and the roots of comfrey have long been used externally as poultices. The material should first be boiled, to sterilize it and to soften it, then mashed to a pulp, cooled to a temperature the patient can bear, and bandaged to the affected part. These poultices have been used with reported success on fresh wounds and old ulcers, boils, carbuncles, infected punctures, and swollen bruises. The allantoin content and the emollient action of this soothing, mucilaginous plant may be enough to explain why these poultices seem to help, but they have been so widely used and reported so uniformly successful in healing such diverse complaints that I am beginning to think that comfrey may have some antibiotic activity that has hitherto been unsuspected. I highly recommend that those scientists who are now searching for antibiotic substances in higher plants (see page 212) take a long, hard look at both the leaves and the roots of common comfrey.

11. Nature's Vitamin Pill:

THE COMMON BLUE VIOLET

(Viola papilionacea)

EVERYONE knows the common blue violet and welcomes it as a beautiful little harbinger of spring, but did you know that this common wildflower can make a contribution to your health? I first suspected that the violet might have hidden nutritional treasures when I saw the children of my Pennsylvania Dutch neighbors avidly eating violet blossoms in the spring, and found that their parents included violet leaves in the wild greens that they cooked and served to their families as a spring tonic. I gathered supplies of both the leaves and the blossoms and had them analyzed. To the best of my knowledge, this was the first time that this common plant had ever been explored nutritionally. The results, as you can see by consulting the chart on page 271, proved that the leaves and the blossoms are amazingly rich in vitamin C, and that the leaves are an excellent source of vitamin A. Translated into common parlance, these figures mean that a small, half-cup serving of violet-leaf greens will fortify your body with as much vitamin C as you could get from four average oranges and also give you more than the recommended minimum daily requirement of vitamin A. The Pennsylvania Dutch children are wise in eating violet blossoms, for these tasty little flowers are three times as rich in vitamin C, weight for weight, as oranges.

This common wayside plant is so familiar that it does not need a description. Unlike many wildflowers, the violet is not harmed by picking its blossoms, for these showy flowers seldom or never produce seed anyway. Apparently they are produced out of sheer exuberance, so take all of them you want, for the more you pick the more the plant will give. Later on, the plant will produce, down under the leaves, some inconspicuous blooms that have no petals and never open, but these are the fruitful blooms, and they bear an abundance of seed.

Although the vitamin content of the violet plant was unknown until I had it analyzed, it has long had a prominent and well-established place in herbal medicine. Violets were frequently mentioned by Homer and Virgil, and apparently they were used by the Athenians in preparing medicine to "moderate anger," to "procure sleep," and to "comfort and strengthen the heart." Pliny wrote that a garland of violets worn about the head would dispel the fumes of wine, preventing drunkenness and hangover. Ancient Britons steeped the blossoms in goat's milk and applied the infusion to the face as a cosmetic that was supposed to increase the beauty of the complexion. An old Anglo-Saxon record lists violets among the herbs that were supposed to be powerful against wicked spirits. Throughout the Middle Ages, violet preparations were used to treat a host of different illnesses, and Violet Syrup still appears in the British Pharmacopoeia. Altogether, the violet seems a very good plant to have around.

My own experiments have proved that violets are not only healthful but can be made into products that are delightful to the taste and beautiful in color. Violet Jam is a luxury product, easy to make, and because it is uncooked, it preserves all that rich vitamin content of the fresh flowers. You will find picking violets for culinary or medicinal use much less tedious than picking them for corsages and flower arrangements, for we want only the blossoms without the stems. Where they are growing thickly you can often use your hand like a cranberry scoop, letting the stems slide between the fingers and pulling off a dozen or more blossoms at each grab. Put as many blossoms as you can pack into a 1-cup measure in your electric blender, add ¾ cup of water and the juice of 1 lemon, and blend until you have a smooth, violet-colored paste. Slowly add 2½ cups of sugar, and blend until you are sure it has dissolved. Stir one package of powdered pectin into ¾ cup water, bring to a boil, and boil hard 1 minute. Pour this hot mixture into the blender with the other ingredients and blend about 1 minute, then quickly pour into jars and seal. This jam will keep in perfect condition for about three weeks

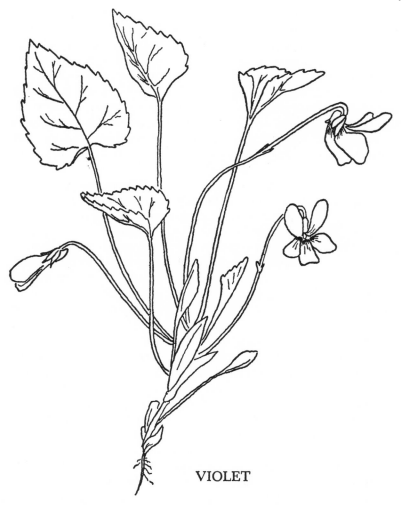

VIOLET

just stored in the refrigerator, but the jars you want to save for next winter must be kept in the freezer.

Violet Jam is not intended to be eaten in great gobs, on toast, as one uses ordinary jam. I like it in little dabs on vanilla wafers, served with tea. It has the characteristic flavor and color of fresh violets, tamed down a bit by the sugar and lemon. I thought I had originated Violet Jam until, on studying the old herbals, I discovered that an almost identical preserve, called violet sugar, or violet plate, had been sold by apothecaries during the reign of Charles II. This violet plate was taken, not only as a sweetmeat, but as a remedy for all chest complaints from bronchitis to consumption, and one ancient writer says it "has power to ease inflammation, roughness of the throat, and comforteth the heart, assuageth the pains of the head and causeth sleep." It would be hard to think of a more pleasant way of taking herbal medicine than eating Violet Jam. It has the sugar-coated pill beat by a mile. Add to the virtues listed above the newly discovered high vitamin content of violets and we see that this is, truly, a noble jam.

The Violet Syrup mentioned above is easily made at home. It is still occasionally prescribed as a very gentle laxative, even milder than prune juice, but it finds its chief medicinal use today as a coloring and flavoring agent to mask unpleasant tastes in other medicines. Unlike most flowers, the violet will give up its coloring matter to a hot-water infusion. Fill any size of glass jar with violet blossoms, cover with boiling water, put a lid on the jar, and let the blossoms infuse for 24 hours. Next day, open the jar and strain the blue infusion, discarding the spent violets. To each cup of the violet extract add the juice of ½ lemon and 2 cups of sugar. Bring to a boil, pour into sterilized jars or bottles, and seal or cap.

When you add the lemon juice, the infusion will turn from blue to purple or reddish. This color change demonstrates another peculiarity of the violet. On the addition of any kind of acid, the blue infusion turns reddish, and on the addition of an alkali, such as baking soda, it turns green, then later, yellow. By using an infusion of standard strength and devising a proper color chart, one could use violets, like litmus paper, to determine the pH of any liquid. Violets have actually been used for this purpose in Europe.

The ancient herbalists had great faith in the healing properties of Violet Syrup and prescribed it to cure ague, epilepsy, pleurisy, quinsy, jaundice, consumption, insomnia, and inflammation of the eyes. Of course, I can't guarantee that Violet Syrup will cure all of that long list of illnesses, but it does have undoubted demulcent and expectorant properties, and I have found it a pretty good cough syrup taken undiluted, a teaspoonful at a dose. However, it tastes so good that I seldom think of it as a medicine; I just let it cure my ills, incidentally, as it tickles my appetite. The syrup is exquisitely beautiful, a clear violet color, and it combines the tastes of sweet, sour, bitter, and aromatic, in just the right proportions to be delightful. It is a pretty good syrup on a pancake, and a couple of spoonfuls over a hot, broiled grapefruit is utterly delicious and extremely decorative.

I like Violet Syrup "on the rocks." Put two or three ice cubes in a tall glass, add 2 tablespoons of violet syrup, then fill the glass with water and stir. It is a beverage that delights the eye as well as the taste buds. To make a Violet Sherbet with a distinctive Oriental air, just stir Violet Syrup into newly fallen snow until the color and consistency are pleasing. A Pakistani guest who tasted this instant sherbet at my home swears that an identical ice is sold in his native land.

To make a beautiful Violet Confection, and one that tastes as good as it looks, empty the contents of a package of lemon gelatin dessert mix into a mixing bowl, add 1 tablespoon of unflavored gelatin, mix well, then add 1 cup of boiling water and stir until all is dissolved. Then pour in 1 cup of Violet Syrup, stir once more, then pour into a wide, shallow dish and chill. Next day cut the stiff jell into small cubes, pile them on your best-looking candy dish, and serve as a special treat.

Violet Jelly is even better-tasting than Violet Jam, and certainly there is no more beautiful jelly in existence. To make it, infuse the flowers just as you do when you make Violet Syrup, and to 2 cups of the infusion add the juice of 1 lemon and 1 package of commercial powdered pectin. Bring this just to a boil, then add 4 cups sugar. Bring back to a boil and boil hard 1 minute, then pour into glasses or jars and seal.

It is not absolutely necessary that you get the curative powers of violet blossoms in sweets. You can make a Violet Aspic Salad that fairly shouts of spring with violet blossoms, and it will be pretty enough to grace any table in the land. Soften 1 tablespoon of unflavored gelatin in ½ cup cold water, then add 1 cup boiling water and stir until it is dissolved. Add 2 tablespoons sugar, ½ teaspoon of salt, and ¼ cup of lemon juice, and stir again. Chill until it just begins to thicken. Now add ½ cup of diced cucumber, ½ cup of sliced radishes, ½ cup of chopped scallions, and 1 cup of violet blossoms. Pour into a fancy mold that has been rinsed in cold water. Chill until firm, then unmold on a bed of wild watercress. You can also beautify and fortify almost any tossed salad by adding 6 to 8 fresh whole violet blossoms to each serving. These can be either incorporated in the salad, where they will blend with the other flavors, or arranged on top of each serving as an unusual and perfectly edible garnish.

Now that we have practically exhausted the uses of violet blossoms, let's turn to those even more healthful violet leaves. These have a richer vitamin C content than any domestic green vegetable known, and they are also an excellent source of vitamin A. But Violet Greens are not only good for you, they are surprisingly good when cooked and served like spinach. Gather only bright-green leaves while they are young and tender. Wash them thoroughly to remove any clinging sand, then, holding a bunch of the leaves in one hand, snip them into ¼-inch shreds with a pair of kitchen shears. Add very little water and cook them in a covered pot for about 15 minutes. Season with salt and butter, and eat the juice and all, as this juice is likely to contain some of the minerals and vitamins. Some of the violet flavor, and even a hint of violet fragrance, are found in the cooked leaves. They also have an herby, spinachy taste and are very slightly astringent.

Another good way to cook Violet Greens is to cook first about 3 slices of bacon until it is crisp. Remove the bacon and dump into the fat about 2 cups of shredded violet leaves. Cover and cook slowly for about 15 minutes, removing the cover only when they need stirring. Taste and add salt if necessary, then garnish with thinly sliced hard-boiled egg, a little raw onion chopped fine, and the crisp bacon crumbled fine.

You can also combine violet leaves with other wild greens that are in season at the same time. They blend exceptionally well with the wild members of the mustard family, such as barbarea, wild watercress, peppergrass, shepherd's-purse, and just plain wild mustard. If you find that you dislike the very slight astringency of cooked violet leaves, try mixing the cooked, chopped Violet Greens with a can of cream of mushroom soup thinned with a half-cup of cream or rich milk. This is an excellent creamed vegetable, and the milk completely eliminates any astringency.

One word of caution: like all intensely green vegetables, violet greens may prove to be slightly laxative to some people. Eat small servings until you determine your tolerance in this respect. With their high vitamin C and vitamin A content, even small servings of

Violet Greens will give the members of your family just the spring tonic they need to help resist the infections so prevalent during that changeable season of the year.

Externally, the leaves have long been used in compresses, plasters, poultices, and ointments. For a violet poultice cover 1 cup of the leaves with boiling water and let stand until cool enough to apply to the affected part. This has been recommended for boils, carbuncles, old wounds, and swellings. The warm leaves are loosely bound to the affected part and changed every few hours.

To make a violet ointment, melt 1 ounce of lanolin and 3 ounces of cocoa butter in a small stone jar. Add as many fresh violet leaves as the melted fats will cover, set in a medium oven, 350°, for 1 hour, pour through a strainer to remove the spent leaves, and store in covered jars. This is a good old-fashioned herbal remedy that is reputed to aid the healing of sores on both man and beast. As one old-time herbalist wrote, 'The violet is a fine pleasing plant of Venus, of mild nature and in no way hurtful."

12. The Fragrant Wild Mints

(*Mentha* species)

THE *Labiatae*, or mint family, is a large one, and some of the most wonderful herbs mentioned in this book, such as sage, pennyroyal, wild thyme, catnip, and ground ivy, belong to this order of plants, but in this chapter we are considering only the true mints, the members of the species *Mentha*, with emphasis on the two best-known members of this fragrant tribe, wild spearmint and wild peppermint. Since ancient days, these two have been among the most famous and highly appreciated of all medicinal and flavoring herbs.

The pious Pharisees of biblical days paid tithes of mint, so this herb was highly esteemed many centuries ago. This mint was probably strewn in the temple to "make a sweet smell before the Lord." In Greek mythology the hospitable Baucis and Philemon scoured their bare wooden table with green mint before laying upon it the food with which they unknowingly entertained divine guests.

(Philemon and Baucis were a pious old couple who lived in Phrygia. At one time the gods Zeus and Hermes disguised themselves as wayfarers and traveled through that country. All the richer people turned them away hungry, but when they came to the house of Philemon and Baucis they were hospitably received. This old couple scrubbed their board with fragrant mint and set out such plain fare as they had—a pitcher of milk and a loaf of bread. Their divine visitors performed a miracle and caused the bread to continue to be the same size loaf of the most delicious bread, no matter how many slices were cut from it, and the pitcher always remained full of the sweetest of all milk, no matter how many glasses were poured from it. As punishment for all the inhospitable people about, these gods caused a flood, but saved Philemon and Baucis. Their cottage was turned into a temple, and they were made priest and priestess of it. At their own request they ended their lives at the same moment, for they loved one another so well that neither could face life without the other. They were turned into two great trees that are supposed still to stand together on the shores of a lake in Phrygia.)

Pliny, the 1st-century naturalist, writes, "The smell of mint stirs up the mind and appetite to a greedy desire of food." An ancient English herbalist writes, "The smelle rejoiceth the heart of man, for which cause they used to strew it in chambers and places of recreation, pleasure and repose, where feasts and banquets are made." Another of the same period refers to mint as "a singularly goode herb," and says, "Being smelled into it is comfortable for the head and memory."

The ancient uses of many herbs have been forgotten, and their use has declined, but this is certainly not true of the mints. We make a more varied and much wider use of mints today than was ever made in any previous period of history, adding it to hundreds of commercial medicines and remedies, using it to flavor candies, chewing gum, toothpaste, cough drops, and dozens of culinary preparations, and adding its cooling effects to face lotions, throat sprays, shaving cream, and cigarettes. The chief difference between our use of the mints and that of the ancients is that where we use extracts, derivatives, and preparations of mint, they used the freshly picked plant, and there they had the better of it, for none of the processed products of mint have ever quite equaled the wonderful flavor, fragrance, and health-giving properties of fresh green mint.

Since spearmint and peppermint were not original natives of America, I suspect that potted mint plants were brought over on the *Mayflower*, for there are some very early references to wild mint in New England. These early immigrants quickly adapted to American conditions and became so thoroughly naturalized that wild spearmint and wild peppermint are now found in damp places throughout the United States.

Wild spearmint, *M. spicata*, can be found in wet places, along roadsides, near small streams, in low meadows and pastures, and in

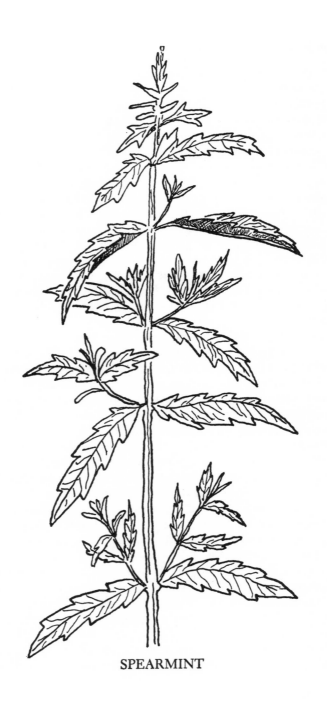

SPEARMINT

cultivated ground nearly everywhere, sometimes even becoming a troublesome weed. It grows in dense patches that are often quite extensive. The individual plants are unbranched, 10 to 20 inches high at maturity, with square, smooth stems, purple or green in color. The leaves are smooth, bright green, one to two inches long, oblong or ovate-lance-shaped, unevenly toothed on the margins, and set on the stem in opposite pairs. The flowers appear in July or August and are usually pale purple, though they are quite variable in color, ranging from almost white to a rather deep purple, with all the plants in one cluster tending to have blossoms of the same shade. These flowers are borne on a crowded terminal cluster, or flower spike, that tapers almost to a point, usually flanked by two auxiliary clusters, one on each side of the main spike, giving the top of the blooming plant a cross-shaped appearance. The individual flowers are tubular, remotely trumpet-shaped, enclosing two long and two short stamens. This is the mint of juleps, mint jellies, and mint sauce.

Peppermint, *M. piperita*, has considerable family resemblance to spearmint, having the usual square stalk, opposite leaves, and pale-purple flowers. The leaves are longer in proportion to their width than spearmint leaves, and they are evenly, rather than unevenly, toothed and slightly rough underneath, rather than being perfectly smooth. The flowers are borne on leafless terminal spikes in loose, disconnected whorls, and the spikes do not taper to a point as do those of spearmint. The easiest way to distinguish these two mints is by the flavor, peppermint being more pungent and having a taste of menthol, which spearmint does not have. Peppermint grows in the same kind of habitats as does spearmint, and is even more common.

It is worth while to search out and taste a sample from all the patches of mint you can find in your neighborhood, for they do not all taste alike. Not only does this herb exhibit wide seedling variation in flavor, but the various mints often hybridize, producing many puzzling forms. On an old abandoned road in the woods, near my place, grows some of the finest wild spearmint I ever tasted, with a fruity flavor and a clean mint taste that is a delight to the tongue. A mile away, on the banks of a small stream, grows some peppermint that has just the right mixture of pungency, mint flavor, and cooling properties of menthol to be perfect. On the other hand, the wild spearmint that grows by the stream just across from my house is very poor in flavor, and I know a whole pasture that is infested with a kind of peppermint that has a very disagreeable weedy taste. If the first sprig of wild mint you taste doesn't exactly delight you, don't thereby conclude that you dislike wild mint. Keep searching, and eventually you will find a mint that is exactly tailored to your tongue.

To list all the uses of the mints would be impossible, as these are easily the most widely used of all the aromatic herbs. There are confections, culinary preparations, and beverages by the score, and home remedies by the dozen, that make use of mint. One herbalist of old England lists more than 40 different illnesses that he claims are successfully treated by mint preparations. These range from stomach ache and seasickness through neuralgia, rheumatism, and lumbago to colds, influenza, and childbirth fever. Strangely, modern medicine still uses certain derivatives of mint in treating many of these same illnesses. The medicinal properties claimed for mint include: stomachic, carminative, stimulant, calmative, diaphoretic, febrifuge, local anesthetic, and disinfectant.

Actually, mint is even more wonderful than the ancient herbalists thought it to be. Unknown or only dimly suspected by them was the fact that fresh mint would also cure scurvy, night blindness, and the great host of illnesses, complaints, and symptoms that arise from dietary deficiencies in vitamins A and C. I had three samples of wild mint analyzed for these vitamins and found that the freshly picked plant had, on the average, approximately as much vitamin C as the same weight of oranges, and more carotene, or provitamin A, than do carrots, making this herb an excellent source of both vitamins.

Despite its great medical reputation, I prefer to think of mint as food rather than as medicine, and indeed, if one is to benefit from its rich vitamin content, the fresh herb must be eaten, not processed into medicines. I would much rather prevent these illnesses by eating proper food than have to cure them with even such a pleasant remedy as mint. I'll let the doctors decide when therapeutic doses of mint preparations will alleviate or cure certain diseases, but I'll bet they never find such an illness in me while fresh mint is in season.

How can one eat enough mint to make it a significant factor in one's daily vitamin intake? It is easy; not only easy, but exceedingly pleasant. We think of mint as a mere flavoring or garnish, adding a sprig of fresh mint to a glass of iced tea or crushing a few leaves in a mint julep, but in the Near East mint is considered primarily a salad plant. I was introduced to mint salads by a Christian Arab from

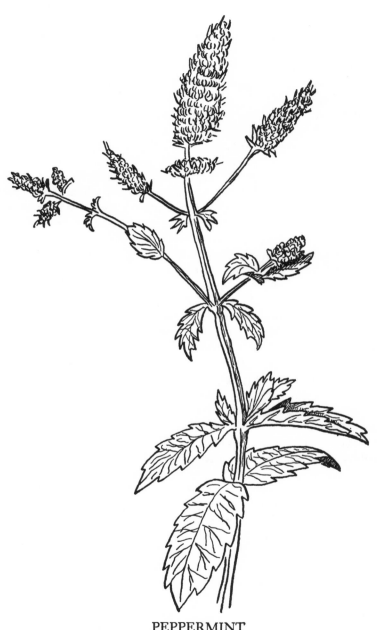

PEPPERMINT

Israel, who used mint as the main ingredient to compound some of the best salads I have ever tasted. There is no recipe. Just add a quantity of fine-chopped mint to almost any tossed salad, for it seems to combine with all salad materials. It must be chopped very fine, and the salad must be thoroughly tossed, for it is unpleasant to get a mouthful of mint alone, but don't be afraid to add enough mint. When it is tempered by oil and vinegar and mingled with the flavors of other greens, it takes at least a half-cupful of chopped mint to properly flavor a big bowl of salad.

Even better is Mint Aspic. Into the jar of your electric blender put the juice of 1 lemon, ½ teaspoon of salt, ¼ cup of sugar, ¼ cup of water, and 2 envelopes of unflavored gelatin. Let stand a few minutes until the gelatin has softened, then add 2 cups boiling water, turn on the blender, and, running it at high speed, gradually add 2 packed cups of fresh mint. Blend until smooth, then pour into a large mixing bowl and set in the refrigerator. Now, here's the trick: Watch that stuff in the bowl, and when it will barely mound when spooned, stir it well and pour into a mold that has been rinsed in cold water. If you happen to let it get a bit too stiff, just set the mixing bowl in warm water and keep stirring the aspic until it reaches a semiliquid consistency. This final stirring is to mix the blended mint evenly throughout the aspic. Otherwise it tends to float to the top. When the aspic has thoroughly set, and you are ready to serve it, dip the mold in hot water for only a second or so and it will slip out easily.

The only thing I can find to object to in this aspic is its yellowish-green, "muckle-dun" color. To correct this, I sometimes cheat a bit and add a few drops of green food coloring at the final stirring. A very small serving of this tasty aspic will give you more than your minimum daily requirements of vitamins A and C. I like to serve it in slices, each slice decorated with some cherry tomatoes cut in half and a few sprigs of watercress. Such a salad, served with perfectly browned broiled lamb chops and some tiny new potatoes and sweet green peas fresh from the garden, will make a dinner that is unexcelled in beauty, tastiness, and wholesomeness.

Almost every cook knows to serve Mint Sauce with roast leg of lamb, but you have never eaten a perfect Mint Sauce until you taste one that is made of freshly picked wild spearmint prepared about an hour before it is to be eaten. Into your electric blender put the juice of ½ lemon, a scant half-cup of water, 2 tablespoons sugar, and 1 packed cup of freshly picked wild spearmint. Blend at high speed until perfectly smooth, chill in the refrigerator for about an hour, stir, and serve with roast lamb or veal. Mint not only provides a wonderful flavor that seems made to go with lamb or veal, but is said to aid greatly the digestion of the crude albuminous fibers of these immature meats.

Mint Jelly is beautiful to look at and sprightly to taste, and can be eaten with meats at lunch or dinner or with toast at breakfast. Avoid all mint jelly recipes that direct you to boil the mint. Boiling mint gives off a wonderful aroma that will pleasantly perfume your kitchen, but this sweet smell means that the volatile flavors and aromas will be missing from your jelly. In a 3-quart saucepan with a dome-shaped lid put 2 cups of freshly picked mint and crush it thoroughly with a potato masher. Add 2 cups of boiling water. Now, invert the saucepan lid and fill it with cold water, adding a couple of ice cubes to keep it cold. Put the saucepan on the heat and bring the water just to a simmer, then remove from the heat and allow it to steep for 10 minutes, keeping it covered with the cooled lid all the time. This rig works like the drip still described in my rose chapter. The volatile flavors, esters, and aromas that ordinarily escape into the air strike the cold lid, condense, and drip back into the infusion. You will hardly be able to notice the smell of mint in the air.

Strain, and to 2 cups of the infusion add ¼ cup of cider vinegar, 4 cups of sugar, and just enough green food coloring to tint the syrup a light emerald green. Stir until the sugar has completely dissolved. Dissolve 1 package commercial powdered pectin in ¾ cup water, bring to a boil, and boil hard 1 minute. Stir this pectin solution into the mint syrup, then pour into glasses and seal.

I use tall thin jars that hold about one cupful each, and pour them only half full, being very careful to pour the jelly carefully so no bubbles appear on the top. When this jelly has set, I take a tiny sprig of fresh mint and set it into the jelly in the exact center of each jar. I then make another batch of mint jelly in exactly the same way and fill the jars, leaving the beautiful little sprigs of mint plainly showing through the jelly. This jelly should be stored in the freezer.

While Mint Jelly is very decorative, a real mint-lover will prefer the flavor of Mint Jam. My uncooked Mint Jam incorporates the whole mint plant and not only captures all the flavor and therapeutic value of fresh mint but also keeps its considerable vitamin content intact, and it is easily made. Put 2 cups of fresh wild mint in your blender, add ½ cup of cider vinegar, ½ cup of water, and 4 cups sugar. Blend until smooth and until all the sugar has dissolved. Dissolve 1 package of powdered pectin in ¾ cup of water, bring to a boil, and boil hard 1 minute, then pour this hot mixture into the blender with the other ingredients and blend on slow speed for 1 minute. Pour it quickly into jars and seal, for unless you move swiftly it will begin to jell in the blender. Again, it is the brownish-yellow-green color that I object to. If this color bothers you, add a few drops of green coloring just before the final blending. This jam should be stored in the freezer. It is our favorite condiment to use with roast leg of lamb during the winter when fresh mint is not available.

Mint Tea has long been a prime remedy for colic, upset stomach, nausea, chills, colds, and influenza, but it is far too good a beverage to be considered only a medicine. I have found that children invariably like Mint Tea if it is presented to them only as a flavorful drink and not as a remedy. It takes quite a lot of fresh mint to make a good tea, about a cupful of the chopped herb to a pint. Cover the chopped herb with 2 cups boiling water, let it infuse for only 5 minutes, then strain. Longer infusion will make a stronger tea, but unfortunately it also becomes weedy tasting. It is a light-amber color with a pronounced aroma and flavor of mint. Serve it with a squeeze of lemon and a little sugar. Besides its medicinal benefits and good taste, this tea probably carries a considerable jolt of water-soluble vitamin C to prevent deficiency diseases and fortify the system against infection.

A good Mint Tea can also be made of the dried herb. Gather the wild mint on a dry day and spread on newspapers in a warm room until it is dry enough to crumble. Store in tight jars to prevent the escape of volatile flavors. Use a tablespoonful of the crumbled herb for each cup of tea, and make it exactly as you make Oriental tea. This tea is said to be a very good remedy for hiccoughs, and one herbal says it is "a sure and certain cure for giddiness." What a find! Let's start a campaign to make this the national drink of our present crop of teen-agers.

In all the concoctions mentioned above, spearmint or peppermint can be used interchangeably. Each kind will give a different product, but both will be pleasing.

There are several other wild mints worth noticing. Horse-mint, M. longifolia, resembles peppermint in size and form, but the flowers are on single, long terminal spikes, and the whole plant is generally covered with fine white hairs. Water-mint, *M. aquatica*, has roundish leaves that are covered with a fine white down; otherwise, it closely resembles the other mints in form, flavor, and fragrance. Native mint, *M. arvensis*, is the only mint that was originally native to the United States. It is found across the northern half of our country and can be distinguished from the naturalized mints by the way it bears its tiny, bell-shaped, light-purple flowers in circles about the plant stem, just above each pair of leaves. It has more the flavor of pennyroyal than of mint, but is still a good herb. It is sometimes smooth, but more often the whole plant is hairy. All of these mints can be used like peppermint or spearmint in home remedies and food products, but each will impart a different flavor.

13. Beating the Cats to the Catnip

(Nepeta Cataria)

CATNIP is another welcome European immigrant that has settled down here to make itself completely at home in American soil and among American flora. Originally a very useful garden herb, it early escaped from confinement and has become a common wild plant about old houses and farmsteads, and, alas, its many uses have almost been forgotten. It is a member of the mint family, a fact betrayed both by its structure and by its aroma. The root is perennial, and early in the spring it starts sending up square, erect, branching stems that may eventually reach a height of three feet. These branching stems are very leafy and covered with a mealy down. The leaves are heart-shaped, minute to three inches long, coarsely toothed at the margins with rounded teeth and covered with a close heavy down, especially on the undersides. This whitish down gives the whole plant a grayish, hoary appearance. The small, two-lipped flowers grow in dense whorls near the summit of each branch, the color being pale pink with tiny purple spots; the anthers show bright red inside each tiny flower.

The most remarkable thing about catnip is the strange fascination this plant has for members of the cat family, not just the domestic cat, but all felines from great lions and tigers down to tiny civets. Rocky Mountain trappers are able to lure the wily lynx just by baiting their traps with a few drops of oil of catnip. Once I tossed a few sprigs of catnip into a cage containing two mountain lions and thor-

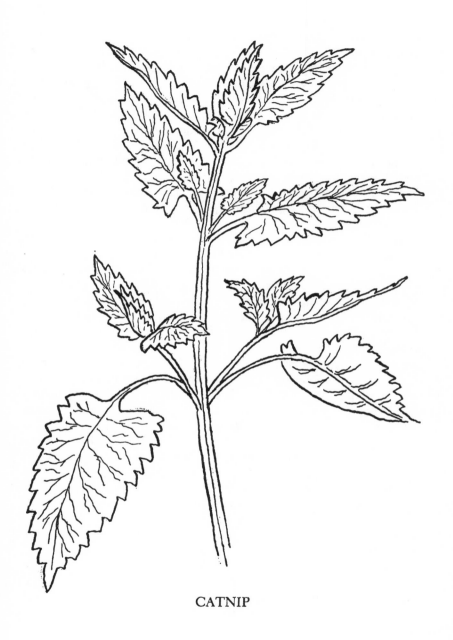

CATNIP

oughly enjoyed the resulting show. They would rub their whiskers against the catnip on the floor of the cage, then roll over and over in it, seemingly trying to cover their whole bodies with its aroma, giving every evidence of being in a kind of ecstasy, both purring like a pair of power lawn mowers. At another time I sprinkled some chopped catnip among a group of playing kittens who had never encountered the plant before, and suddenly their playfulness was accelerated by a factor of ten. They dashed about the room at full speed, some going in one direction, and some in the other. This resulted in many head-on collisions, each such accident knocking both kittens across the room. However, nothing seemed to hurt or daunt them, and each one would leap up and resume the wild play as if nothing had happened.

Catnip grows all about the old farmhouse in which I live, so that my cat lives in a junkie's paradise. He is hopelessly addicted to catnip and goes out several times a day to get his "fix." He has favorite clumps, and always returns to these rather than to any others. He will sit with his head inside the clump inhaling the stimulating aroma, occasionally biting on a leaf, not eating it but merely bruising it with his teeth, then rubbing his whiskers in the exuding juice. If I approach him at this time, he will set up a strange querulous cry, for he is not a do-it-yourself-er at heart, and he has learned that if he begs in a pitiful tone I will crush a handful of fresh catnip and rub it all over his fur. Then he will roll on the ground, purring loudly and making happy little noises in his throat. If I can ever discover an herb that affects me as catnip seems to affect cats, I will disappear into a herbal limbo of ecstasy.

Besides making cats ecstatic, catnip has a long history of use for many purposes by human beings. The tea habit was deeply ingrained in the English people long before the first tea was imported from Asia, decoctions being made of many wild and domestic herbs. Catnip was one of the favorites among these country teas, and it had its advocates even after the introduction of Oriental tea, many claiming that Catnip Tea tasted better and had all the good effects of commercial tea without its harmful stimulants. Besides drinking it for pure pleasure, it was widely used in several domestic remedies, taken for a great variety of complaints. Even officially, catnip has been listed in various pharmacopoeias and dispensatories to relieve gastric distress, as a tonic, mild stimulant, nervine, antispasmodic, and to reduce fever, and stimulate the menstrual flow. What more could you ask of one plant?

My Pennsylvania Dutch neighbors know the catnip plant simply as "tea," and they swear by the decoction made from the dried leaves. They take cold Catnip Tea before meals as a tonic, to stimulate jaded appetites, and hot Catnip Tea after meals, to prevent gas. They take the hot tea at bedtime as a soporific, to insure a good night's rest, a practice much safer and more wholesome than the habit of taking tranquilizers and sleeping pills, and certainly far less expensive. This catnip nightcap is also reputed to be a sure cure for nightmares. When any member of the family gets a cold, or the flu, he is put to bed, covered warmly, and given hot Catnip Tea with lemon. This is said to induce copious sweating, lower the fever, and help break up the cold. In view of recent research on reputed cold cures, it is doubtful that this treatment ever measurably shortens or actually cures any cold, but it does make the patient more comfortable and helps him to rest, and I defy any cold medicine to do more. Also, making this tea and serving it at the bedside gives other members of the family an opportunity to express their love and concern in a material way, assuring the patient that he is cherished and that those about him genuinely want to help him get better. These things are important, too.

Some of my neighbors use hot Catnip Tea both as a warming drink in winter and as a cooling drink in summer. This is not as illogical as it sounds on the first reading. After being chilled by exposure, they drink a cup of hot Catnip Tea to "warm their insides" while sitting before the fire to warm their outsides. Hot water would probably do as much, but would not be nearly so pleasant to take. They also consider this warming draught a prophylactic against colds. Who can say when a cold has been prevented? Until some dedicated scientist sets up a rigidly controlled experiment, giving hot Catnip Tea to large numbers of people after each exposure, over a considerable time, and refusing it to an equally large control group, we cannot estimate how many colds can be prevented by this practice. However, in view of the considerable vitamin content of catnip, it seems logical that it might help to build up resistance to infection and thus actually prevent some colds.

In summer, aficionados claim that a cup of hot Catnip Tea will help them to cool off when they have become overheated. This, too, can be explained. Catnip is said to promote sweating without appreciably raising the body temperature. The light, loose clothing people wear in summer allows the air to circulate freely around the body, quickly evaporating this extra perspiration and rapidly cooling the skin surface. The Dutch in the East Indies used gin in the same way and claimed that it was a far more efficient cooler than any iced drink. It is merely a trick to induce the body's natural thermostat to turn on the cooler.

As an emmenagogue, to correct a scanty or suppressed menstrual discharge, some juice expressed from the fresh leaves, rather than the tea, is used. This is taken, a tablespoonful at a dose, three times a day, until the condition is corrected. Despite the many virtues they assign to Catnip Tea, I suspect that the main reason my neighbors make so much use of it is that they like it. They learn to like it very early in life, one neighbor assuring me that warm Catnip Tea is the surest cure for colic in babies, and that a little sweetened Catnip Tea will act as a mild nervine, or soothing syrup, to pacify a fretful child. I have seen small children wad their jaws with fresh catnip leaves, then slowly masticate this cud as they went about their play, swallowing the juice their teeth expressed. I have tried this and find the taste bitter-aromatic, a bit strong, but not really unpleasant, and I found it easy to learn to like it. Now, during the season that fresh leaves are available, I am almost constantly chewing catnip as I work around the yard and garden, and I have become almost as hopelessly addicted to it as my cat is, but I must admit that it doesn't seem to do as much for me as it does for him.

As with many other herbs used in domestic remedies, I wondered how many of the benefits ascribed to it were due to the nutrients it contained. Since it is a member of the mint family, with very dark-green leaves, I suspected that catnip might be rich in vitamins and had it partially explored. The gratifying results appear on page 271, and you can see it returned an excellent yield of A and C, the only vitamins for which it was tested. Quite likely it also contains other beneficial vitamins and almost certainly some of the essential minerals. It is probably just as good for children to chew catnip, which they have learned to appreciate, as it would be for them to take the handfuls of capsules loaded with synthetic vitamins that many children are forced to swallow each day, and it is certainly cheaper. The girls usually stop this catnip-chewing habit about the time they stop playing in the fields and woods and start going with the boys, while the boys early graduate to chewing tobacco. However, by this time they have acquired a taste for catnip that will make healthful Catnip Tea a welcome beverage for the rest of their lives.

Gather catnip about the time the first blooms appear, in July, and dry it in a warm, dry place. Again, it is my hot attic that seems the ideal dehydrator. I merely spread the catnip stalks on newspapers there and find it perfectly dried in about a week. When it is thoroughly dry, crumble but do not powder the leaves and remove all large stems. Pack the tea in tight containers and store in a dry place. Use a little more dried catnip than you would ordinary tea for the same amount of water. Just pour the boiling water over the dried leaves and let it steep a few minutes. The flavor and aroma of catnip are very volatile, so this herb should never be boiled. Always make this tea in a tightly covered vessel, and if you use a metal tea ball and make it right in the cup, a good way, then cover the cup with the saucer while it is brewing.

The fragrance of Catnip Tea is reminiscent of mint, but it also has a characteristic aroma all its own. When used as a carminative, to aid digestion, present it in demitasse cups at the end of the meal, each serving garnished with a thin slice of lemon. Another excellent way to use catnip as a carminative is to serve Candied Catnip Leaves instead of commercial after-dinner mints. The flavor of lemon goes so well with catnip that I worked out a way of candying catnip leaves that takes advantage of this fact.

To make Candied Catnip Leaves, select medium-sized catnip leaves that are free from insect damage. Thin the white of 1 egg with the juice of 1 lemon, not beating it together, but merely gently stirring until the egg and lemon are thoroughly mixed. Dip each catnip leaf in this mixture, then sprinkle both sides with granulated sugar. Allow to dry for at least one day before use, and if the candied leaves are well dried, then kept in a tight container in the refrigerator, they will stay perfectly fresh and tasty for weeks.

All in all, I think catnip is an herb well worth knowing. With its high vitamin content, good taste, and pleasant aroma, and the many benefits it is reputed to confer, I think it a shame that we are beginning to allow catnip to become a monopoly of cats.

14. Those Healthful Heaths

BEARBERRY, BEAR'S GRAPE, OR KINNIKINICK

(*Arctostaphylos Uva-ursi*)

THE BEARBERRY is disappointing as a fruit, but it makes one of the most effective of all home remedies for kidney, bladder, and other urinary troubles. This ground-hugging shrub is found in northern regions around the world, growing in sandy, sterile soil and on gravelly ridges in Europe, Asia, and North America. On this continent it grows in suitable situations from the Arctic Circle south to Virginia and Missouri, around the Great Lakes, and on westward to the Pacific.

Bearberry is a true shrub, and the branched stems are woody, but weak and flexible; though they may reach a length of two feet, they lie flat across the ground, often forming extensive mats, and even the branches seldom rise more than three inches. The evergreen leaves are about one inch long, leathery, with a glossy green upper surface and lighter underneath, shaped like a spatula with a wider, rounded outer end and tapering toward a short leafstalk. The pretty, waxy flowers are urn-shaped, reddish-white or white, and appear in clusters of from three to fifteen at the ends of the branches. These are followed by bright-red berries, currant-size, smooth, glossy, and attractive. They have tough skins enclosing an insipid mealy pulp that has five hard seeds.

Like all plants that have been important in herbal medicine and have entered deeply into folklore, the bearberry, or bear's grape, has a host of common names, most of them assigning this rough, poor-

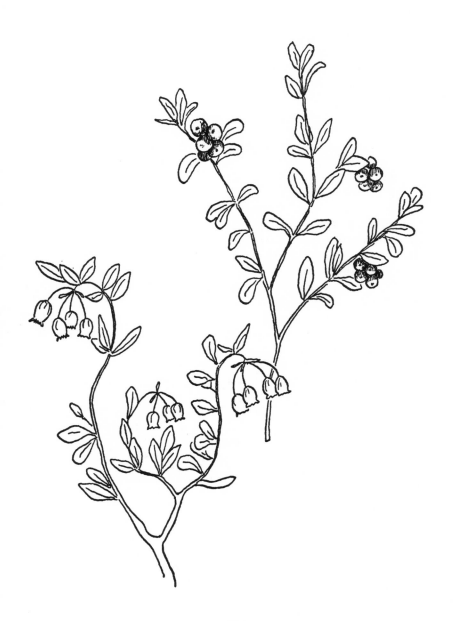

BEARBERRY

flavored fruit to bears, boars, crows, foxes, or some other wild animal. The botanical name for the genus, *Arctostaphylos*, is Greek and means "bear's grape." The specific name, *Uva-ursi*, is Latin and also means "bear's grape," so when I say the name of this plant is "bear's-grape, *Arctostaphylos Uva-ursi*," I'm really saying that its name is "bear's-grape, bear's-grape, bear's-grape," which is getting downright ridiculous.

Bearberries are barely edible raw, being nutritious and mildly medicinal but wholly uninviting. They are dry, mealy, slightly astringent, and almost tasteless. Cooked, they are a little better.

I once gathered a quantity of these berries in the barrens of New Jersey and made them into a Bearberry Marmalade. I first simmered the berries about 20 minutes in enough water to cover, then rubbed them through a sieve to remove the tough skins and hard seeds. I then peeled 1 orange and 1 lemon, shaved off about half of the white part of the peels, clipped these peels into fine shreds with a pair of kitchen shears, and boiled them in about a cup of water for 15 minutes. While the peels were cooking, I divided the orange and lemon into sections, then carefully removed all seeds and chopped them into fairly coarse chunks. When the peels had boiled long enough I drained them and added the chopped fruit and 2 cups of the strained bearberry pulp. This mixture was returned to the fire and simmered for 10 minutes more. Then I stirred 1 package commercial powdered gelatin into the fruit, and as soon as it regained a hard boil I added 5 cups of sugar. When it had regained a boil and boiled very hard for about 3 minutes, I ladled it into 7 straight-sided ½-pint sterilized jars and sealed with sterilized dome lids.

This marmalade tasted excellent to me. My wife, who is my sternest critic when it comes to wild foods, pronounced it very good, then practically ruined her compliment by remarking that it would probably have been even better if I had left out the bearberries. Oh, well, we can still keep in mind that bearberries have considerable food value and could serve as a survival food in emergencies, even if they don't taste very good.

As a medicinal plant, bearberry has won recognition not only from herbalists but also from the medical profession. Until recently, it appeared in most of the world's pharmacopoeias, and it is still recognized as having real therapeutic value by our own *U.S. Dispensatory*. The medicinal part of bearberry is the leaves, and these should be gathered in early autumn; reject those that are insect-eaten or otherwise imperfect. Being so thick and leathery, these leaves are a bit difficult to dry. A good way is to spread them on an old window screen—one layer deep, so air can get at all sides—and dry them in a warm room.

These dried leaves are astringent, tonic, and diuretic, and have an antiseptic effect on the urinary passages. The manner in which this remedy works is quite interesting. Certain constituents of bearberry leaves combine with chemicals normally found in the urine to form hydroquinone in sufficient quantities to be a potent germ killer in the urinary tract. Bearberry is given for cystitis, nephritis, urethritis, or, in more common language, any infection of the plumbing. An interesting side effect that should occasion no alarm is that while taking bearberry infusion the urine sometimes turns a bright-green color.

Bearberry leaves give up their medicinal virtues to both alcohol and boiling water. The best way to prepare the infusion is to put an ounce of the dried, crumbled leaves into a jar and pour on enough gin (another diuretic) just to cover them. Let them soak in the gin overnight, then next morning pour on a pint of boiling water and let the leaves infuse until cool. Strain, and take the entire amount in one day, in three equal doses, morning, noon, and night. I have not had an opportunity to observe how well this works on urinary infections, but it seems to be a reasonable and scientifically justifiable remedy, and is apparently harmless, as I took a pint of this infusion every day for a week with no untoward results beyond a slight diuretic effect.

WINTERGREEN OR TEABERRY
(*Gaultheria procumbens*)

This tiny plant is also called checkerberry, boxberry, partridgeberry, mountain tea, woodsman's tea, ground holly, and probably 15 or 20 other common names in various parts of its range, which extends from Maine to Georgia and west to Minnesota. This proliferation of common names indicates how much the fine aroma and sweet taste of this little plant have been appreciated, and how extensively it has entered into local herbal lore and folk medicine.

Wintergreen is a shrubby, recumbent plant with a slender, extensive stem that creeps just on or just under the surface of the ground.

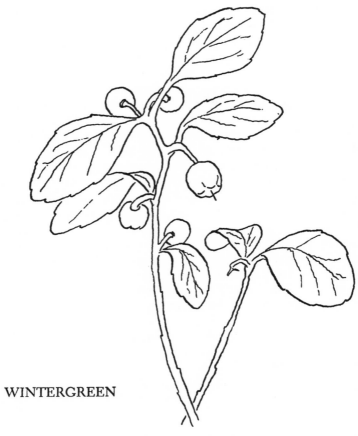

WINTERGREEN

The little leafy flowering and fruiting sprigs that we think of as entire plants are really branches from the creeping stems. These little fruiting branches stand only three to six inches high, with a few leaves clustered near the top. Mature wintergreen leaves are stiff and rigid, 1 to 1½ inches long, oval in outline, glossy green above and lighter below, sometimes tinged with red or purple, and one finds entire leaves of a bright-red color. The margins of these leaves are finely toothed, with the teeth bristle-tipped. The white, bell-shaped, nodding flowers, about ¼ inch across, are solitary, on recurved stems that spring from the axils of the leaves. As the plant matures, the white corolla falls off, and the green calyx gradually becomes fleshy and round, turning into a berrylike fruit about ¼ inch in diameter and becoming bright red in autumn. The leaves are evergreen, and even the bright berries that hang on the plant all winter if unmolested often are plumper and sweeter when the snow melts than they were in the fall.

The flavor and aroma of wintergreen are familiar to all Americans, as it is often used to flavor cough drops, candies, chewing gum, and toothpaste. The wintergreen flavors used by medicine and industry are almost all made synthetically, and even when it is a natural flavor, it does not come from the wintergreen plant but is usually distilled from the bark and twigs of the sweet birch, *Betula lenta*, which, by some strange natural coincidence, contains exactly the same fragrant essential oil that is found in wintergreen. Commercial distillers use birch because it is cheaper and easier to gather in quantity.

I have known and loved the wintergreen plant for years, but I must admit that it took a long time for me to find much use for it. Its chief value to me was that it so often gave me an excuse to escape from my typewriter and go wandering in the woods. No other plant has led me into the woods so often. From my study window I can see a hill covered with an open forest of mixed pines and hardwoods. Beneath the trees grow mountain laurel, wild azaleas, rhododendrons, and scads of squaw-huckleberries and blueberries, and beneath these shrubby plants the ground is literally carpeted with wintergreen. The wintergreen is in season all year round, and in midwinter I have kicked away the snow and gathered a few of the tasty, spicy leaves and sometimes found one or two of the brilliant-red berries. The berries are not squashy, so I carry a supply in my pocket to nibble as I stroll through the woods. Both the berries and the leaves have the warm familiar flavor of wintergreen, so if I can't find berries, I eat the young leaves, preferring those that are bright red.

My Pennsylvania Dutch neighbors like Wintergreen Tea, so I have often tried making it of both the fresh and the dried leaves. The flavor has been pleasant enough, but so faint as to be barely detectable. Children love it with milk and sugar, but I have noticed that children also love plain hot water with milk and sugar. My own son liked this hot-water tea, and when he was first learning to talk he would clamor for "hot-otter tea" whenever the grownups were having tea or coffee. My complaint about Wintergreen Tea, made from either the fresh or dried leaves, has always been that it tasted altogether too much like "hot-otter tea."

It was purely by accident that I finally learned the proper way to make Wintergreen Tea. I kept trying to add more leaves to get more strength, until one day I filled a quart jar to the top with freshly picked leaves, then filled the jar with boiling water. Even this much wintergreen produced a beverage with a flavor too weak to be at all exciting. For some reason, after tasting a spoonful of it, I didn't throw it out, but covered the jar and left it in the warm kitchen. My wife has become used to herbal experiments going on all over the house and has learned not to toss out any concoction that she comes across, no matter how unlikely-looking it may be, so the jar of water-covered wintergreen leaves stayed there. A day later I noticed some bubbles rising in the jar, indicating that some kind of fermentation was going on. I tasted the liquid and was agreeably surprised to find the winter-green flavor much stronger than it had been when I first made the tea. I let it bubble for another day, then heated the covered jar in hot water and poured out a cup of the tea. Purely from color-choice I had gathered only bright-red leaves, and the tea was a beautiful pink color. It had a pronounced, but still pleasant, wintergreen flavor and a delightful hint of pungency that warmed my mouth and throat and even gave a warm glow in my stomach, similar to that experienced after taking a shot of neat whiskey. Here was a Wintergreen Tea that spoke with authority!

I wanted to know why this bland beverage had suddenly come alive after a little fermentation. It wasn't because it had produced ethyl alcohol, for alcohol was undetectable in the finished tea. I searched further into the scanty literature on this herb and finally discovered that away back when wintergreen flavoring was actually made of wintergreen, the manufacturers of this essence steeped the winter-green plants until they had undergone some fermentation before distilling the essential oil. I learned in my search that Gaultheria oil, the flavoring substance of wintergreen, exists in only minute quanti-ties in the fresh plant, but is developed by fermentation.

Wintergreen Tea is usually taken purely for its pleasant spicy taste, its slightly stimulating effect, and as a warming and restorative hot beverage. When used as a medicine, it used to be given for head-aches, the aches and pains of colds and grippe, and especially for rheumatic pains in joints and muscles, for lumbago, gout, and sci-atica. It was used as an antipyretic, or febrifuge, to dispel fever or at least to lower the temperature of feverish patients, and to increase perspiration and the discharge of urine.

Naturally, I was a bit dubious about the benefits of Wintergreen Tea in this long list of illnesses, until I discovered that the essential oil of wintergreen is 99 percent methyl salicylate. It was not until the latter half of the 17th century that scientific medicine discovered the importance of the salicylates as antipyretics, antirheumatics, diaphoretics, and analgesics, useful in allaying aches and pains, thus confirming the empirical findings that the herbalists had discovered centuries before. When the American Indians and those badly maligned "old wives" were giving strong Wintergreen Tea for fever, headaches, rheumatism, and other aches and pains, they were far in advance of the medical science of their day. Of course, modern medicine has at its disposal many kinds of salicylates, each tailored to do a specific job, and no longer has to depend on Wintergreen Tea.

I was elated to discover that I could make a tasty beverage of wintergreen that would also cure my ills. However, unless I kept a batch constantly brewing, any sickness would either disappear or call for more radical remedies before I could get Wintergreen Tea made by this slow process. I did learn to speed it up a little. I found that adding some of the water from a former brew started the fermentation immediately, and the leaves would be ready to make tea in 24 hours, which still fell a bit short of an "instant" tea that could be offered on the spur of the moment. When the fermented leaves were dried they gave a stronger tea than fresh leaves, and also added a little color to the brew, but one still couldn't call it a strong tea. For my own use, I went back to the slow-brewing process, which produces a strong, delightful beverage.

Still in an experimental mood, I took some of the strong tea made of freshly fermented leaves, cooled it, sweetened it to taste, then added a teaspoon of active dry yeast to a gallon of it. In about 2 hours this began to bubble a bit, so I bottled it and capped it tightly. In a week, it was a lively beverage, and when chilled to ice-cold, was like wintergreen-flavored champagne, except that this had no kick that I could detect. I have since offered it to many guests, including children, and while some think it is alcoholic because of the warmth it imparts to the stomach, no one has ever gotten high on it.

Some of my Pennsylvania Dutch neighbors do make a Wintergreen Wine with a good "kick," so I begged a recipe from one of them and experimented with this more potent beverage. It called for

1 gallon of the bright-red leaves of wintergreen. After the tedious job of selecting only the reddest leaves I could find, I put them in a 3-gallon crock and added 1 gallon of boiling water. Next day I drained off the first infusion and saved it, and added another gallon of boiling water to the same leaves. When this had cooled a bit, I added 4 pounds of honey, the infusion I had drained off, and 2 teaspoons active dry yeast, and stirred it all well. I kept the crock covered, but inspected it every day. After about 2 weeks, I could discern no further activity, so I carefully decanted off the wine and put it in clean bottles, capping it tightly with crown caps. After a few months I opened a bottle, purely from scientific interest, and found it slightly sparkling, with a beautiful pink color and a clean, wintergreen flavor.

My Dutch neighbors consider this a wine for women and invalids, and I have heard of quilting bees that became hilarious parties when Wintergreen Wine flowed a bit too freely. When one of my neighbors had the flu, I took him a bottle of this pink wine, and he remarked that it was medicine like this that made being sick worth while.

I tried making Turkish-style paste of nearly every herb mentioned in this book, but wintergreen was one of the few that produced a confection that I felt I could recommend. Make Wintergreen Candy from strong wintergreen tea, brewed from freshly fermented leaves. Mix 1 package unflavored gelatin with ¾ cup of sugar. Add ½ cup of cooled Wintergreen Tea and stir until the sugar is all dissolved, then add a cup of very hot Wintergreen Tea and stir again, until the gelatin is all dissolved. Pour into a small, straight-sided pan, and set it in the refrigerator until the next day. Dip the pan in warm water for just an instant, then shake it to loosen the jelly, and pull it out of the pan onto a cutting board. Cut into cubes, and it's ready to eat. It will keep for a week or more in the refrigerator, so you can offer it to later guests. It has a pronounced wintergreen flavor, and a hint of cinnamon-like pungency that is very good.

Naturally I was not content to let those bright-red wintergreen berries remain no more than a pleasant nibble to be enjoyed on walks through the woods. I tried making cooked jams and preserves of them, but all these concoctions were dismal failures. The heat necessary to make such preserves drives off all the wintergreen flavor, leaving the berries tasting exactly like nothing at all. Finally, with the help of a blender, I worked out an uncooked Wintergreen Jam that preserved all the fresh flavor and aroma and was a delight to the nose and the tongue, yes, and with its pretty pink color, it was also a delight to the eye.

In the jar of a blender I put 2 cups of bright, fresh wintergreen berries, the juice of 1 lemon and 1 cup of strong Wintergreen Tea. This was blended until smooth and evenly pink-colored, then poured into a mixing bowl and mixed with 4 cups sugar. In a small saucepan I combined 1 package commercial pectin and ¾ cup of water, brought this to a boil, boiled hard for 1 minute, then stirred it thoroughly into the berry mixture. This was stirred until I was sure I had it all evenly blended together, then quickly ladled into small sterilized jars, sealed, and stored in the refrigerator. By the next day it had jelled beautifully, and for those who enjoy wintergreen flavor, the taste was very fine. If you intend to keep this jam more than a month, you'd better store it in the freezer, where it will keep indefinitely.

I had often wished that I could make the berries attractive as a nibble to offer party guests, but when glacéed in the usual manner, these berries, which have very little acid, lacked character. Finally I invented a new Wintergreen Glacé Syrup that gave the berries a bright, polished look and added tang to their taste. In a small saucepan mix 1 package of unflavored gelatin with ⅔ cup of sugar. Add ¼ cup water and the juice of 1 lemon. Stir well, then let it set for 5 minutes, so the gelatin will soften. Place on medium heat and bring just to a boil, then remove. Spear each wintergreen berry with a toothpick, dip it in the syrup, and stick it upright in a chunk of Styrofoam to harden and dry. If the syrup starts to coagulate in the pan while you are doing this, float the utensil in warm water to keep the syrup liquid. Although this is enough syrup to coat thousands of wintergreen berries, I'm sure you won't want to do so many at one time. But you can put it into a small jar and store it in your refrigerator, and when you want to use it again, it can be liquefied by warming it over hot water.

A piece of Styrofoam, or even an apple, stuck full of toothpicks bearing bright, polished wintergreen berries, makes a nice decoration on a party table. The lemon juice adds the needed acid to make these small red berries something special. Even if wintergreen had no medicinal value whatever, I would continue to use it purely for the joy it has been able to add to my life. The enjoyment of the bounty of nature has a health-giving effect quite apart from the drug content of the herbs we use, for joy itself is more curative than any medicine in the doctor's book.

15. Ground-Ivy or Gill-over-the-ground

(Glechoma hederacea)

THIS recumbent little relative of catnip is very common in lawns, in shady, damp places, along waysides, and around the edges of woods. It is easily identified by the supine, square stems, the opposite, rounded, kidney-shaped leaves, which are downy, green on both sides, with rounded teeth on the margins, and borne on short leaf-stalks. These leaves range in size from minute to more than one inch across, and the whole plant seldom rises more than six inches above the ground unless supported by adjacent vegetation. The upper few pairs of leaves are often purplish, and in the axils of these upper leaves the purplish-blue flowers are found, three or four in a cluster. The flowers begin blooming about the end of April, and one can find plants in bloom until the winter freeze-up.

It is often said that one can judge how deeply a plant has entered folklore by the number of common names by which it is called. If this is true, then ground-ivy has entered deeply, for besides the two names given in the heading of this section, it has been known as Robin-run-up-the-hedge, alehoof, Lizzie-run-in-the-hedge, hedge-maids, tunhoof, haymaids, cat's-foot, field balm, and a host of other names equally peculiar. I'm sure that had I been born in rural England I would have been called Theophilus-run-in-the-woods, or Euell-pick-by-the-hedgerows.

Ground-ivy has long been known, not only in England, but all over Europe; it has followed man wherever he has gone, and is now naturalized over most of the civilized world. It was early introduced in America and has made itself thoroughly at home, crowding out other plants in every suitable habitat. It was well-known in ancient Greece and Rome, and even then was highly regarded as a medicinal herb When Greek physicians were fashionable in ancient Rome, Galen and Dioscorides, two of the most learned of these Greek doctors were both high in their praises of the healing properties of this herb. Its popularity persisted through the Middle Ages, and Gerard, the 16th-century English herbalist, claims Discorides for his authority when he recommends ground-ivy for "ache in the hucklebone." He also extols its virtues for a host of other illnesses, then adds, almost as an afterthought, "It also purgeth the head from rheumatic humours flowing from the brain."

How's your hucklebone doing these days? You'd better watch those "rheumatic humours" flowing from your brain! Ever since reading Gerard's statements, my wife has always been willing to make me a fresh cup of Gill Tea, for she insists that the kind of humor that flows from my brain badly needs curing.

Ground-ivy has long been discarded from the official *materia medica,* but this does not mean that it is useless or harmful. To be efficacious, ground-ivy must be freshly picked, and one can hardly expect a modern physician to stop by the roadside and pick his own medicine. Modern pharmacology is not interested in ground-ivy, nor in any other botanical that must be used the same day it is picked. Drug manufacturers today want something that can be dried and powdered, extracted and bottled, or otherwise preserved so that it can be stored, shipped, accurately measured, and sold at a profit. Ground-ivy simply doesn't fill the bill.

It would be hard to support many of the ancient claims about the curative powers of ground-ivy, but it would not be hard to defend it as an excellent home remedy. Primarily, it is used as a bitter tonic, as a nutritive tea, and as an excellent remedy for stubborn coughs. Its most time-honored uses are as an antiscorbutic and to prevent "painter's colic," which is a euphemism for lead poisoning. Both these uses point to a high vitamin C content, as synthetic vitamin C is the modern, scientific treatment for both these conditions today. When I recently had ground-ivy investigated for its vitamin C content, it proved to be an excellent source of ascorbic acid. (See page 271.)

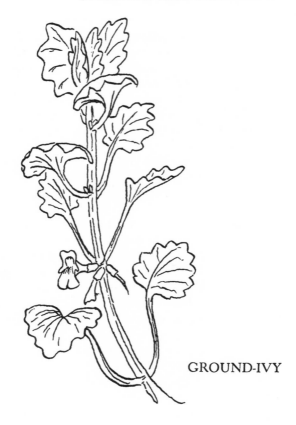

GROUND-IVY

Here is another example of the herbalist using the right remedy long before scientific medicine discovered that it *was* the right remedy.

The best way to take ground-ivy is as Gill Tea, which is an infusion of the freshly picked plant. Use ¼ cup of the chopped whole herb for each cup of tea. Cover with boiling water and keep it covered while it is brewing, to keep the volatile materials from escaping. If it is being given for a cough due to a common cold, and the patient is in bed, give it very hot, sweetened with honey, a cupful four times per day. If it is being given for a stubborn cough, and the patient is up and about, give one wineglassful of the cold infusion, sweetened with honey, four times per day. The reason for the difference in temperatures is that hot Gill Tea causes sweating, which might be beneficial if the patient is in bed and well covered, but might have the opposite effect if he is up and exposed to drafts or breezes.

To use ground-ivy as a Bitter Tonic, just chill unsweetened Gill Tea in the refrigerator and sip a glassful of it, very slowly, about a half-hour before breakfast. The taste of all these concoctions is aromatic-bitter, with a bit of herbiness. Just as some sweets are more palatable than others, and some sours taste good and others indifferent or bad, so there are bitters and bitters. To my taste, ground-ivy furnishes a good bitter, and a small wineglassful of the infusion, taken ice-cold, half an hour before breakfast, stimulates my taste buds, tones my stomach, and gives me an excellent appetite for that important meal. My wife sometimes joins me in this eye-opener, but she mixes her ground-ivy infusion with orange juice to improve the taste. For me, this addition of orange juice defeats the purpose of the bitter tonic. Even unsweetened orange juice contains considerable natural fruit sugar, and this sugar content spoils my appetite instead of stimulating it. However, my wife, who is watching her weight, claims that she needs no appetite stimulant, and since orange juice adds vitamins A and C to the drink, she takes it as a natural vitamin concentrate.

Those who are exposed to possible lead poisoning, such as painters, and those who handle lead-bearing agricultural sprays, should take four wineglasses of cold ground-ivy infusion per day, and when used for this purpose the addition of orange juice would be advantageous, as it would increase the vitamin C content. When the body is well supplied with vitamin C, any lead that is accidentally introduced into the system combines with this vitamin and is harmlessly excreted through the kidneys. If vitamin C is not present, the lead accumulates, and if one is continuously exposed to it, it can soon reach dangerously poisonous levels. Of course, the vitamin C is destroyed in the process of eliminating unwanted lead, so the supply must be continually renewed. Those exposed to lead contamination have a far higher vitamin C requirement than do people not so exposed.

The old books say that the expressed juice of fresh ground-ivy, snuffed up the nose, is a sure cure for headache. This juice was also used for bruises, such as black eyes. If a little got into the eye, apparently no harm was done, for the infusion was also recommended as a wash for "sore or weak eyes." When the green plant was bruised and applied as a poultice, it was reputed to cure such horrors as "abscesses, gatherings, tumours, fistulas, hollow ulcers, and green wounds." The juice was even dropped in the ears to cure "the humming noise and ringing sound ... and for them that are hard of hearing."

Before the introduction of hops into England, ground-ivy was used to clarify beer and to improve its flavor and keeping qualities. It was from this use that it acquired the common names, *alehoof* and *tunhoof*, the beer being fermented in huge casks called "tuns." Even the name "gill" probably comes from the French *guiller*, meaning "to ferment beer." After the introduction of hops, ground-ivy was still used to cure "sick" beer, that is, beer that had become cloudy or discolored. Culpepper, the British herbalist, writing in the 17th century, says of ground-ivy, "It is good to tun up with new drink, for it will clarify it in a night that it will be fitter to be drank the next morning; or if any drink be thick with removing or any other accident, it will do the like in a few hours."

I haven't tried brewing my own beer with ground-ivy, but my Pennsylvania Dutch neighbors make an herb wine of it and other bitter herbs, which they hold in high repute as a tonic and appetizer. A recipe that was given to me after I had complimented the product goes like this: One pint ground-ivy, use the whole herb; 1 pint dandelion leaves; 1 pint chicory leaves; 1 pint burdock leaves; the rinds of 5 lemons; 5 tangerines; and 5 oranges (what, no grapefruit?). Put these ingredients, unchopped, into a large kettle, bring to a boil, then barely simmer for 1 hour. Strain into a stone jar or "crock" and add 2 pounds of brown sugar. Spread a cake of soft yeast on a slice of toasted rye bread and float it on top of the mixture. Be careful to let it reach a temperature of just lukewarm before floating the yeast, for yeast is a living product and can be killed by high temperatures. Cover with a cloth and allow to ferment. For some reason this wine ferments slowly, so don't try to rush it. Leave it in the crock until it stops bubbling and clears. This could be in about 2 weeks, sometimes a few days more or less. As soon as it clears, siphon it into clean bottles and cap tightly with crown caps. Use amber or green bottles, for light penetrating clear glass bottles will debase the flavor, making it taste "skunky." Age it in the dark for about 3 months before broaching it. You will find that it has a clear, beautiful, greenish-amber color and is slightly lively, like champagne. The taste is intensely bitter, but it is a clean-tasting bitter that sets your saliva and gastric juices to flowing. It is not intended for heavy tippling, but is used solely as a bitter tonic and appetizer. An ounce glassful, half an hour before eating, will make you ravenous. Give several wine-glasses a day to those whose appetites are jaded.

While I would not quite go along with Gerard in saying, "It [ground-ivy] is proved to be the best medicine in the world," I would join Culpepper in saying, "It is a singular herb for all inward wounds, and . . . [expels] melancholy by opening the stoppings of the spleen."

16. The Wild and Woolly Horehound

(Marrubium vulgare)

I HAVE enjoyed the flavor of horehound for as long as I can remember. I did not know that this musky, bittersweet flavoring came from an herb; I merely accepted it as another of the delightful flavors the mysterious and wonderful world offered to a small boy with pennies to spend at the candy counter. I never thought of it as a medicine, but considered it a favorite confection and thought a cough was a small price to pay for the privilege of sucking on horehound drops.

When I was six years old, my family moved to a farm, and there, just outside the fence that surrounded our backyard, was a clump of woolly white plants that my mother told me were horehound. I was immensely excited and wanted to use this herb immediately. We gathered a handful of the fresh leaves and my mother took them into the kitchen and made some hard horehound candy while I dogged her every step and absorbed the whole process. I didn't quite believe this weedy-looking herb could produce the flavor to which I was addicted, until Mother poured the candy into a buttered plate and handed me the pan to scrape, but there it was, the same fascinating, musky bittersweet, and even better than horehound candy from the store. Now, nearly fifty years later, I can recapture that happy moment by merely nibbling on a fresh leaf of horehound.

Horehound is not a very decorative herb. It is low and woolly-white, with a number of squarish stems springing from a perennial root each year, and seldom standing more than a foot high. The leaves are round or oval, much wrinkled, toothed at the margins, and covered with a dense, felted wool that gives the whole plant a downy, whitish appearance. The flowers are small, mintlike and white, and are borne in whorls just above each pair of upper leafstalks. The most certain identification feature is the taste, this flavor being instantly recognizable by anyone who has ever sucked on a horehound drop.

Horehound is a member of the mint family, and, like many of our wild herbs, is not really a native, but was introduced by herbalists from Europe. It easily escaped from herb gardens and seems perfectly able to maintain itself in the wild. It actually seems to prefer poor, dry soil, so that it frequently establishes itself where there is little competition from native flora. I have seen wild horehound growing in many parts of the United States, from coast to coast, but was unable to find any near my present home in the lush countryside of central Pennsylvania. A few packages of horehound seed soon remedied that situation, and now "wild" horehound grows in many places in my neighborhood.

Unlike most mints, the flavor and medicinal properties of horehound are not volatile or easily lost, so the plant can be used fresh or dried, and can be boiled without driving off the flavor. To dry horehound, gather it, stems and all, and spread on papers in a warm room until it will crumble easily. Crumble the leaves, remove all large stems, and store the herb in closed jars. To use fresh horehound, merely gather the leaves.

To make a strong horehound infusion, boil 1 cup of fresh leaves or ¼ cup of dried herb with 2 cups water for 10 minutes, let it sit for about 5 minutes more, then strain. This is too strong to be drunk as tea, but 1 part infusion and 2 parts boiling water make a horehound tea that many enjoy as a pleasant beverage, and it is a common household remedy for coughs and colds. Given very hot to a patient who is in bed and warmly covered, it will induce sweating, which many believe to be beneficial during a cold. It will also help to allay coughs and ease any tickling of the throat, enabling the patient to rest easier, and the fact that you are there administering potions, spreading blankets, and fussing about shows the patient that his welfare matters to you. Don't tell me that home remedies are useless!

To make a pleasant-tasting and efficacious cough syrup, mix 1 part horehound infusion with 2 parts honey and stir until it is smooth. This sounds like an awful lot of honey, but if you use less, the cough syrup is likely to spoil. I use thyme honey in making this cough syrup, thus getting the medicinal benefits of two fine herbs, but ordinary clover honey will make a good syrup.

To make Horehound Drops, use 1 cup horehound infusion, made as directed above, to 2 cups white sugar. Put the sugar in a small but deep saucepan and stir in ⅛ teaspoon cream of tartar, then add the horehound infusion. Stir until the sugar has dissolved, then cook over low heat until it reaches just 290° on a candy thermometer, or until a drop in cold water will become a hard, glassy ball. Pour on a buttered plate and score into cough-drop sizes when it has half hardened. When cool, break apart and keep in a cool place until used.

Horehound heals in gentle and harmless ways, containing no drastic or dangerous drugs. The dosage is not critical, and it can be freely given to children or weakened patients. Horehound preparations are easily made and pleasant to the taste. I consider horehound an ideal herb for use in home remedies.

AMERICAN PENNYROYAL OR SQUAW MINT
(Hedeoma pulegioides)

American pennyroyal is a sweet-smelling herb that makes one of the most flavorful teas of any wild plant. It has a very extensive range, being found from New England to the Dakotas and southward to Florida and Texas. It likes a dry, sterile, acid soil, and where such conditions prevail it is likely to be abundant. Just back of my house begins a trail that leads to a maze of deer trails and abandoned logging roads that thread miles of uninhabited woodland. For some reason, pennyroyal finds these unused and slightly overgrown trails and roads an ideal place to grow. I often walk these paths through the straggly, second-growth timber looking for herbs, berries, or nuts, or sometimes just walking, with all senses attuned, ready to receive any new lesson that nature can teach me for that day. In summer one often comes on places where these roads have let a little sunshine in, and pennyroyal grows so thickly there that each step will crush a dozen plants, filling the air with their sweet perfume.

This is a native American plant and not to be confused with the European pennyroyal, *Mentha pulegium*. Our pennyroyal is a small, branched annual, six to twelve inches high, and, as in all members of

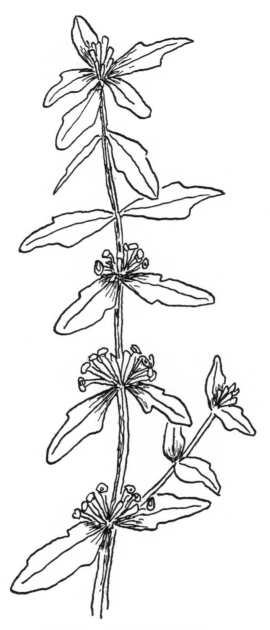

AMERICAN PENNYROYAL

the mint family, it has square stems and opposite leaves. The leaves are small, oval, and toothed at the edges. The pale-violet flowers are quite small and appear in the axils of the leaves in midsummer. Gather the herb in June or July and dry it in a cool room, for too much heat drives away some of its flavor and fragrance. When dry, store the herb in tightly sealed fruit jars so that none of the flavor can escape. Make the tea just as you make regular tea, using about a teaspoonful of the herb for every cup of tea wanted. Do not boil pennyroyal, or you will have a very fragrant kitchen but a flavorless tea.

Pennyroyal tastes good enough so that you need no other excuse for drinking it, but it is also reputed to have many medicinal virtues. It is considered a mild stimulant, aromatic, diaphoretic, carminative, and emmenagogue. It earned its alternate common name, "squaw mint," because it was used by Indian women to help suppressed menstruation. Some Cherokee and other Southwestern Indians have claimed that if a woman drinks plenty of hot pennyroyal tea regularly, she will not become pregnant. I doubt that this will challenge the oral contraceptive, but it might bear some investigation.

Pennyroyal is not, however, a monopoly of females, for this tea, besides tasting good, is said to be gently corrective to headaches, nausea, constipation, and nervousness, and, properly administered, very helpful in the treatment of colds, influenza, bronchitis, sinusitis, and fevers. The recommended way to treat the latter group of complaints with pennyroyal is to have the patient sit on the edge of the bed with his feet in a footbath as hot as he can bear it, with a little dry mustard added to the water to make it seem even hotter, and to drink one or two cups of pennyroyal tea as hot as he can stand it. Then tuck the patient into bed, turn the electric blanket up on high, and make him sweat it out.

Finally, pennyroyal is a natural insect repellent. When I am bothered by mosquitoes or gnats out in the woods, I crush a handful of pennyroyal and rub it on all exposed skin. It is about as effective as commercial repellents, and the effect lasts about as long, and certainly pennyroyal has the pleasanter smell. The fresh herb strewn in your doghouse, whether occupied by you or your dog, will keep away fleas. The dried herb, made into sachets and packed away with your woolens, will keep away moths and give your clothes a much more pleasant aroma than they have when paradichlorobenzene moth repellents are used.

17. Common Garden Sage Gone Wild

(*Salvia officinalis*)

IT SHOULD be clear to the reader by now that this is not a book about cultivated herbs. I am no herb grower but a collector of wildings. However, I must admit that in the case of a few desirable herbs I have encouraged them to grow wild where they would be accessible to me. Garden sage is not a native American plant, but it early escaped from gardens and has become somewhat naturalized in many places. I have occasionally found wild sage growing along roadsides, about abandoned farmsteads and in waste places, but was unable to find any growing near where I now live, a situation I decided to remedy. I bought several packages of sage seed and wherever I saw a likely place for sage to grow, on my land or on my neighbor's, I scratched up a bit of ground and scattered a few seeds. The season was good, and this semi-wild sage grew wonderfully. Sage is an evergreen member of the mint family, and now in midwinter I can look out my study window and see a large clump of this "wild" sage poking its leaves above the snow.

There are two European superstitions about sage. One saying is that if sage grows well it is a sign that its planter is thriving financially, and another states that when sage grows luxuriantly it is a sign that the wife rules the household. My own experience would indicate that there may be truth in both these superstitions. Recently, a near neighbor called me on the phone and said, "Didn't you tell me you were hunting for wild sage? Well, I was just walking over near where my place joins yours and I saw several clumps of wild sage I didn't know I had. Come over and help yourself." I thanked him kindly, but explained that I had also found wild sage on my place that I had unaccountably overlooked before.

There are many varieties of cultivated sage, some with red leaves, some with white ones, and some variegated. These arise from natural "sports" or "mutations," and when such oddities are decorative or desirable they can be propagated by cuttings, but they will not come true from seed. Wild sage, which is seedling sage, usually grows about a foot high with wiry, squarish stems and opposite, grayish-green leaves, showing that it is related to the mints. The leaves are one to two inches long, oblong in shape, rounded at the ends, and finely wrinkled by a network of veins that give the leaf surface a mosaic pattern. The flowers appear in May or June in whorls and are purplish in color. All parts of the plant have a strong, spicy odor and a warm, aromatic, bitter flavor.

Sage gets its genus name, *Salvia*, from the Latin word for "save"— an allusion to its many medicinal uses—and *officinalis* indicates that it was on the official list of medicinal herbs. Ancient physicians and the herbalists of the Middle Ages ascribed marvelous healing and preventive powers to sage. Few medicinal herbs were valued more highly. It was reputed to cure agues and fevers, palsy and nervous trembling, dyspepsia and flatulence, biliousness and liver complaints, sore throat and sore, soft gums, tonsillitis and typhoid fever, headache and nervous excitement, and it was a prime remedy for colds in the head. One woman writer says that anyone who takes a wine infusion of sage through the winter months will never show any ill effects from old age but will retain full muscular strength, brightness of vision, and youthful appearance all his days. Another herbalist says that one who drinks sage tea and rinses his hair in it will never get gray, or, if the hair is already gray, this treatment will restore it to its natural color. Some go even further. There was a Latin saying current in the Middle Ages that translates, "Why should a man die when sage grows in his garden?" An old English couplet tells us, "He who would live for aye/ Must eat Sage in the month of May." Sage was even reputed to cure the grief and sorrow of those who had recently had a death in the family, though why anybody should die when such a marvelous medicine was available, I'll never know.

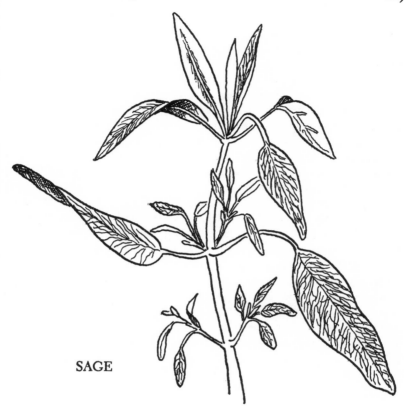

SAGE

I found it impossible to read these glowing accounts of the wondrous preventive and curative powers of sage without wanting to give this magic herb a thorough trial. When I encountered the statement, "Sage is singularly good for the head and brains, it quickeneth the senses and memory—" I knew that sage was the herb for me. And try it I did. I took the prescribed dose of sage wine from the end of September until the end of March; I ate fresh sage leaves every day in the month of May; betweentimes I drank sage tea and rinsed my hair in it, and several times I ate nine leaves every morning for nine days, and fasted an hour after, before eating my breakfast. But alas, this modern sage seems to have lost the marvelous powers possessed by its ancient ancestors. My hair is still gray, my bifocals still perch on my nose, and, while my health is excellent, it is no better than it was before I started on this sage kick.

Sage retained its reputation as a potent medicine until recent times, long after the medical professional had been differentiated from the country herbalist and culler of simples. At first it occupied an honored place in all European and American pharmacopoeias, but was gradually dropped from later editions, disappearing from our own pharmacopoeia last of all. It is no longer prescribed by physicians, and even its use in domestic remedies has almost disappeared. From being considered one of the most valuable remedies in the whole *materia medica*, sage has been gradually relegated to being no more than a well-known culinary herb. Even its culinary use has a medical history. Originally sage was added to sausage, to stuffing for fowls, or to pork dressing, to counteract the tendency of these rich foods to cause indigestion and flatulence. Its health-protecting advantages have been forgotten, but meanwhile we have learned to like its flavor in rich meat dishes. Today, many housewives are really giving their families an herbal remedy when they think they are only flavoring the meat.

Sage deserves a better fate than its present slide into obscurity and disuse. While it is not the cure-all or wonder drug that the ancients thought it to be, very few herbs are. Although it did not restore my lost youth, sage is still a warm, aromatic stimulant, a good-flavored bitter tonic, an excellent astringent, and an efficacious carminative, and as such it should find more use than it does in home remedies. The culinary seasoning is made by drying sage leaves in a warm room and then crumbling them, but the home remedies are best made of the fresh leaves, which can be picked the year round.

My own adaptation of the ancient recipe for that magic Sage Wine calls for a quart of the best claret, a cupful of fresh sage leaves, and, of course, an electric blender. Put the sage into the blender with about half the wine and run it on high speed for about 2 minutes, which will practically reduce the sage leaves to liquid. Pour this wine-sage mixture back into the bottle with the other wine, give it a shake, and cap it tightly. Make enough room in the wine bottle so it will hold the extra bulk of the minced sage leaves. To "keep off all diseases to the fourth degree" and to keep yourself young and beautiful, take 3 tablespoonfuls of the wine with 1 tablespoonful of running water an hour before breakfast every morning. Keep this up from Michaelmas (Sept. 29) until the last of March. Taken at this rate you will consume only about a quart of wine per month, so if you limit your drinking to this tipple no one can accuse you of using this remedy as an excuse for guzzling. After pouring out your daily dose give the bottle a shake, every day, before you put it away.

We may laugh at the claims of the old herbalists about the efficacy of this wine, but there is no doubt that it did ward off some illnesses and cure others when it was popular. You will notice that the time it was taken was during the winter months when fresh vegetables were almost impossible to get, in the days before freezers, canning, or supermarkets. In those days nearly everyone suffered from at least minor vitamin deficiencies almost every winter. Sage is no vitamin giant, but the fresh leaves, which can be obtained all winter, do give good yields of vitamins A and C, probably enough to prevent the worst deficiency diseases. Those who pinned their faith on this wine would probably have been better off had they eaten a handful of sage leaves every day, but drinking sage wine was undoubtedly better than getting no vitamins at all.

Eating sage "every day in the month of May" presents no problem. A few of the leaves chopped fine and added to a tossed salad will give it an aromatic tang that most people like at first taste. The fresh leaves, chopped fine and added to butter or cream cheese, make excellent sandwiches for lunch or teatime. Or you can make the leaves into a tasty confection that everyone, even children, will enjoy in place of regular after-dinner mints. Simply thin a little egg white with a little water—the proportions are not critical—dampen the leaves with this, and sprinkle them with granulated sugar. Let them dry for a day before they are to be served; those left over can be kept in the refrigerator for as long as a month. The country people in the south of England formerly solved the problem of eating sage with a head-on approach, simply chewing up and swallowing nine leaves of sage every morning for nine days, each time waiting at least an hour after taking this dose before eating breakfast. This was supposed to cure ague, trembling, palsy, and fevers, as well as acting as a tonic, stimulating a debilitated appetite, and preventing indigestion. I have tried this and find it not too unpleasant a feat, fresh sage leaves having a more minty and palatable taste than does the dried herb with which we are all familiar.

Sage Tea is reputed to cure a host of ills, including headache, head colds, dyspepsia, delirium, nervous excitement, delayed menses, and lethargy. Even if Sage Tea had no medicinal benefits whatever, I would still drink it for flavor alone, for it is a tasty beverage when brewed from the fresh, green leaves. One reference says that the Chinese thought Sage Tea so good that they would formerly trade many pounds of their own tea for one pound of sage. To make this pleasant drink use ½ ounce of chopped fresh sage leaves, 1 ounce of sugar, the juice of 1 lemon and 1 teaspoonful of grated lemon rind. Pour over all this a quart of boiling water and let it infuse for half an hour, then strain through a cloth strainer. It can either be chilled in the refrigerator and served ice-cold, or be reheated and served hot. I like it either way. Besides all its other virtues, this tea is said to be cooling in fevers and useful to cleanse and purify the blood. I sometimes serve tiny cups of this aromatic herb tea as the last course of the wild-food dinners I frequently give. So far, no one has ever suffered any distress from these "wild parties," but I'm always afraid a dyspeptic guest may someday develop indigestion after such a meal and blame it on the wild food, forgetting that he suffers the same way no matter what kind of food he eats. A little cup of this antiflatulent, digestive tea is not only a charming note on which to end an unusual meal, but it is also a little extra insurance that my wild foods will sit well on everyone's stomach. Can you wonder that I risked being called a fraud and a nature-faker by encouraging "wild" sage to grow in my neighborhood?

18. How to Have a Wild Thyme

(*Thymus Serpyllum*)

WILD THYME is not the same species as *Thymus vulgaris*, the familiar garden thyme, but it is closely related to it and is used for much the same purposes. The ancients preferred garden thyme for culinary use and wild thyme for medicinal remedies. This plant is a native of Eurasia, growing wild from Spain to Siberia, but especially abundantly in the Alps. It was brought to this country by some colonial herbalist and has escaped into many sections of the country, seemingly having no trouble adapting to our climate and soil conditions. In the northern Catskills it is exceedingly abundant, probably outnumbering all other plants in this area.

It is a sprawly, somewhat weedy-looking plant, the squarish stems rather woody but thin and weak, reaching a length of about a foot. The leaves are not as tiny as those of garden thyme, but they are still small, about an eighth of an inch broad and little over a half inch long, and, as in all members of the mint family, they grow in opposite pairs. The redeeming feature of wild thyme, as far as appearance goes, is the flower. The pretty purple flowers grow in a terminal, showy cluster, two to six inches long, the crowded corollas being about half an inch long, making the cylindrical cluster about an inch in diameter. The seeds are abundantly produced, but are so tiny that a quart measure of them would contain more than four million seeds.

According to ancient tradition, if a girl wears a corsage of wild thyme flowers it means she is looking for a sweetheart, and according

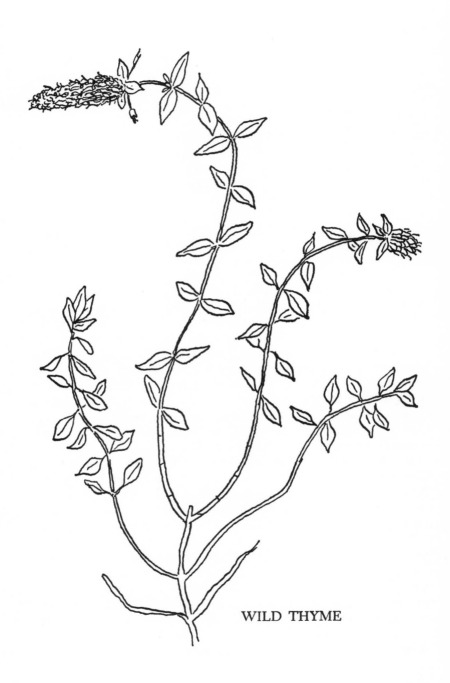

WILD THYME

to another tradition, if a bashful boy drinks enough wild thyme tea it will give him courage to take her up on it. Besides its use to young lovers, wild thyme has from early times been a highly respected medicinal herb, and the honey that bees make from its copious nectar, secreted by the flowers, is considered by some to be the finest of all honeys, not only delicious in flavor but conferring many of the medicinal benefits of the herb, such as relieving a cough, dispelling melancholia, insuring a good night's sleep, and preventing nightmares. It is harmless and wholesome, and hence the dosage is not critical, but an adult should take at least a tablespoonful at a dose for it to be effective. This honey is often offered for sale at farmhouses in the northern Catskills, or you can order it from Walnut Acres, Penns Creek, Pa. Don't expect it to taste like other honeys, for thyme honey has a unique and different flavor, tasting noticeably of the thyme from which it was made.

It is possible to get all the healing benefits of thyme honey from Thyme Syrup made with ordinary honey. Gather the herb while it is in full bloom, and dry it in a warm room. When it is thoroughly dried, crumble and store it in a tight container. To make the syrup pour 1 pint of boiling water over 1 ounce of the herb and allow it to infuse until cool. Strain, to the liquid add 1 cup honey, and stir until it is thoroughly dissolved. Keep in the refrigerator and take 1 or 2 tablespoonfuls several times a day. This is a safe and efficacious remedy for convulsive coughs, whooping cough, catarrh, and sore throat. One of the best and safest of the commercial cough remedies that are sold by the millions of dollars' worth every year is no more than saccharated thyme, and this simple home remedy will do the job fully as well.

An even pleasanter way to take this herb is as Wild Thyme Tea. Use a teaspoonful of the herb to a cupful of boiling water, and make it just as you make ordinary tea. I use a metal tea ball and don't have to bother about straining it. Sweeten the tea with a teaspoonful of honey. Believe it or not, you can use wild thyme to help recover from a wild time. Wild Thyme Tea, sweetened with honey, and with a pinch of salt added to each cupful, is far better to sober up on than black coffee, as it will not leave you jittery and nervous. The next day a few cups of Wild Thyme Tea taken at intervals through the day will help to ease the headache, nervousness, and queasy stomach of the hangover, and will help prevent the sufferer from being tempted to take dangerous sedative drugs, which, while temporarily relieving the symptoms, only delay the recovery.

However, Wild Thyme Tea is not a monopoly of the drinking classes. According to the books, it is aromatic, antiseptic, stimulant, carminative, diaphoretic, antispasmodic, diuretic, and emmenagogic, and thus should be a capital remedy for a wide variety of complaints. Because of its thymol content, Wild Thyme Tea is somewhat antiseptic and will arrest gastric fermentation, making it an excellent remedy for flatulence, wind spasms, and colic. Like the syrup, it is good for cough, catarrh, and sore throat, and in addition it will promote perspiration in feverish colds. It is also reported to be a great reliever of headaches, nervousness, insomnia, and nightmares.

The Romans gave Wild Thyme Tea as a sovereign remedy to melancholy persons. Culpepper tells us, "It is so harmless, you need not fear the use of it." Pliny says that burning some of the dried herb in the house will put to flight all venomous creatures. Like garden thyme, it is a valuable culinary herb, and a pinch of powdered wild thyme will add a new dimension to stuffings, sauces, pickles, soups, and stews. Although it tends to become almost a nuisance in some areas, wild thyme is a weed to be encouraged.

19. Did You Ever
Eat a Pine Tree?

(*Pinus Strobus*)

IT IS popular to speak about the large trees in many parts of the world as the oldest living things, and this is true, but I wonder how many people realize that these "oldest living things" are actually composed almost entirely of long-dead cells. In the most ancient tree, the oldest living cell may be only a few years old. In the trunk of a large tree the only living part is some layers of live cells—outside the wood proper and inside the dry bark—called the sapwood, the cambium, and the inner bark, and all these layers put together may be only a fraction of an inch thick. The living parts of the tree are being constantly renewed, and while a tree may be the oldest living thing, there is nothing in it that is alive that has been so for very long. In the mightiest forest giant, life goes on as it does elsewhere, by abandoning the old and renewing itself in the young.

The living layers of cambium and inner bark on many kinds of trees have often been used in medicine, in home remedies, and even as a source of food. In 1732, when Linnaeus, the father of modern botany, was tramping through Lapland, he reported that the Lapps were largely subsisting on "fir bark." This was from the tree known to us as Scotch pine, *P. sylvestris*. The Lapps gathered large quantities of this bark each spring when the rising sap made it easy to peel it from the trees. They preferred the bark from large trees and thought the bark near the base of the tree the best. They removed the brown outer layer and hung the strips of white inner bark under the eaves of their barns to dry. If food was plentiful the next winter, this bark was fed to their hogs and cattle, and was reported to be very fattening, but if other foods were scarce, the Lapps would grind this dried bark and make a famine bread of it, which was very nutritious, but, to Linnaeus's taste, not very palatable.

It is not usually realized how much the American Indians formerly depended on tree barks for food. Early explorers often reported extensive areas where the bark had been peeled from all the large trees. The eastern Indians favored the barks from the pine family, especially that from the white pine, *P. Strobus*, although the inner barks of other trees, such as black birch and slippery elm, were relished. The Adirondack Mountains, in northern New York, were named for a tribe of Indians who lived in that area, and the word *adirondack* comes from an Indian phrase meaning "tree eaters." Some of the tribes of the Pacific Northwest commonly made a hard bread of the inner bark of the western hemlock, which is not related to the plant with which Socrates was poisoned.

The eastern white pine is one of the largest forest trees found from Canada south to Georgia and west to Iowa, often towering two hundred feet high in terminal or virgin forests. The bark is greenish and smooth on young trees, becoming brown and furrowed on the large, old ones. The needles are a grayish blue-green in color, soft and flexible with no prickles or points, three to five inches long, growing five in a cluster—a valuable recognition feature.

I had no trouble finding white pine bark with which to experiment. I simply inquired at a country sawmill where white pine had been recently cut, drove where they directed me, and peeled the bark from the stumps. White pine bark should always be gathered in May or June, for then it is sweeter, juicier, and easier to peel from the wood. The inner bark must be separated from the dry, outer bark. I tried boiling this fresh inner bark as the Indians did, and it reduced to a glutinous mass from which the more bothersome wood fibers were easily removed. I'm sure it was wholesome and nutritious, but in the area of palatability it left much to be desired. It is said that the Indians cooked this bark with meat, so I tried boiling some with beef, but when I tasted it I felt that instead of making the bark edible I had merely ruined a good piece of beef.

I imagine that one who grew up eating this food, as the Indian children did, would find it good. When I was a boy in New Mexico,

I gathered clear golden drops of resin that had hardened on the piñon trees and used it for chewing gum. It turned a pretty pink color between the teeth, and I enjoyed its piny, resiny flavor. At that time I also enjoyed chewing on the inner bark of ponderosa pine whenever we cut a large tree in spring (the bark peeled easily then). I found this inner bark sweet, juicy, and mucilaginous, and actually enjoyed its piny flavor, but it is apparently not a durable preference, for now I dislike both the resin and the inner bark, finding them to taste too much of turpentine to be good.

I wanted some dried bark for herbal remedies and further food experiments, so I hung some of my strips of white pine bark in a warm attic room until it was thoroughly dry. It still wouldn't grind very well, so I gave it an additional drying in an oven with the door propped slightly open so moisture could escape. The heat caused the bark to swell slightly, and it became a great deal more friable and grindable. The redried bark was cut into small pieces with a hatchet, and ground, about a cupful at a time, in the electric blender. Most recipes for home remedies made of this inner bark call for coarsely ground bark, so I put the pulverized bark through a flour sifter, using the fine part that passed through the sieve for food experiments and the coarser stuff for cough syrup.

The fine powder was a weak yellowish-orange color with a slight odor of turpentine and a taste that was at first very sweet and mucilaginous, but was quickly followed by a disagreeable bitterness and astringency. There is no doubt about this material's being nutritious. It contains sugar and starch, and, according to two U.S. Government sources, it is rich in vitamin C. I hoped the bitterness and astringency would disappear on cooking, but, alas, these tastes are very persistent, and I can't say that the bread I made with it was an unqualified success. I mixed the fine powder half-and-half with wheat flour and followed a recipe for yeast-raised rolls. They were of good texture and perfectly edible, but they also had a disagreeable bitter taste and more than a hint of turpentine flavor about them, and I felt the rolls would have been better without the white pine flour.

Dried white pine bark is still a valuable ingredient in cough remedies. It is an official drug in the U.S. Pharmacopoeia, the National Formulary, and the U.S. Dispensatory. Its medicinal properties are expectorant and diuretic. It is most often prescribed in the title role of Compound White Pine Syrup, or, as the doctor would write it on

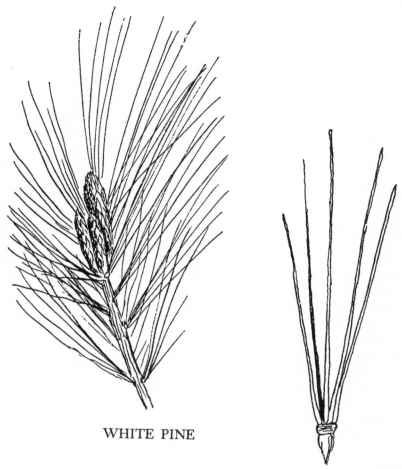

WHITE PINE

your prescription, *Syrupus Pini Albae Compositus*. This is a real
herbal mixture and a good illustration of the fact that modern medicine does not disdain herbal remedies if they are effective. This compound contains not only white pine bark, but wild cherry bark, spike-
nard, poplar buds, bloodroot, sassafras-root bark, and amaranth. If
you want to make this remedy at home, there is a complete recipe
in the *National Formulary*, but I was afraid no amateur herbalist
would ever get all those ingredients together at the same time, so I
have included a much simpler recipe for a White Pine, Whisky, and

Honey Cough Syrup that was given to me by an old herbalist in Indiana.

Put ½ cup of coarsely ground white pine bark in a jar and cover it with ⅔ cup of boiling water. When cool, add ½ cup of whisky, seal the jar, and let it soak overnight, shaking the jar occasionally. Next day, strain it, and to the liquid add 1 cup of honey. Mix until the liquid is homogeneous, and it is ready to use. If kept in a capped or corked bottle, this cough syrup will keep indefinitely without spoiling, and it certainly seems an effective cough remedy. A dose is 1 tablespoonful for adults and 1 teaspoonful for children, as needed.

Other parts of the white pine besides the inner bark are useful. It is reliably reported that the Ojibway Indians formerly gathered the unexpanded aments, or staminate catkins, which often grow in clusters of five or six together near the bases of the terminal shoots on each branch or twig, and stewed them with their meats. These are tedious to gather, for each catkin is less than an inch long and less than a quarter-inch in diameter, cylindrical in shape, covered with soft, light-brown scales, but green and tender inside if gathered while they are still young and firm. These must be very nutritious, for they have a sweet, starchy taste, and judging from their color and origin, I would expect to find rich yields of both vitamins A and C, if they are ever explored for their nutritional constituents. Unfortunately, when I gathered some of them and stewed them in chicken broth they had the same pitchy, piny flavor to which I object in other white pine products. They would make an excellent emergency food, and I would, of course, gladly eat them as an alternative to starvation, but until I become hungrier than I have been recently I would not call them gourmet products.

New Englanders formerly candied the peeled new shoots of white pine, gathered before they became woody. I tried some of these peeled tender shoots, boiling them until tender, draining off that cooking water and then boiling them for 20 minutes in a syrup made of equal parts of sugar and water. The syrup was then drained off, and the candied shoots were partly dried, then rolled in granulated sugar. This paleface delicacy tasted a little more civilized than the savage Indian foods I had been trying, but even this candy was nothing about which I could get very excited. I would have considered it a pretty good-tasting cough medicine, and it would probably help control a cough, but I'm sure I have eaten much better confections.

White pine needles have been tested for nutritional benefits, and they gave good yields of vitamin A and about five times as much vitamin C as is found in lemons. Had those old-timers, who used to suffer from scurvy every winter when fresh vegetables were unavailable, used an infusion of white pine needles instead of tea or coffee, they would never have been touched by scurvy. Pine Needle Tea, made by pouring 1 pint of boiling water over 1 ounce of fresh white pine needles chopped fine, is about the most palatable pine product I have tasted. With a squeeze of lemon and a little sugar it is almost enjoyable, and it gives a feeling of great virtue to know that as you drink it you are fortifying your body with two essential vitamins in which most modern diets are deficient. Judging from taste and effects, I believe all white pine products, the staminate catkins, the tender shoots, and the green needles, have the same expectorant and diuretic properties that make the bark an official drug, and I'm sure a good cough syrup could be made with any of these tree parts if the bark is unavailable.

I have high respect for the medicinal and nutritional properties of white pine products, but you must have gathered by now that I care very little for their taste. Nevertheless, the economic hazards of writing for a living being what they are, I intend to bear in mind that these lordly trees can furnish substantial and nutritious, if somewhat ill-tasting, food in times of need, but the emergency will have to be pretty dire before I consume any large quantity of it. My current taste in food-gathering poses no threat of extinction to the white pine.

There is one pine product that I consider one of the most palatable of all wild foods. This is the piñon nut, which is the seed of two kinds of western pines. The Rocky Mountain nut pine, *P. edulis*, is a small tree not over forty feet in height, and most specimens are far less than that. The trunk is short and the branches low, often sweeping the ground. The stiff, curved needles are only about an inch long and grow two, rarely three, in a cluster, and are very fragrant. The cones are almost globular in shape, about two inches in diameter. They mature the second season, so one can make a fairly accurate estimate of the prospects for next year's piñon crop by observing the number of immature cones on the trees in the fall. The seeds are about a half-inch long and a little less than that in diameter, sometimes very slightly flattened. This tree is characteristic of the dry, mountainous regions of New Mexico, Colorado, and Arizona. The one-leaved nut pine, *P.*

monophylla, is a very similar tree found growing in the dry mountains of Utah, Arizona, California, and Nevada, and is easily distinguished from the above species, since its needles grow singly, rather than as twins or triplets. The nuts of both kinds are equally delicious.

The piñon is not a dependable cropper, and only once in every seven or eight years is there a real bumper crop in any one area. On these good years piñon nuts become a considerable source of income to the Indians, for these nuts command high prices on the market. When I was a boy in New Mexico, I gave the local Indians some competition, for in very good years one could make higher wages gathering piñon nuts than doing any other work that was available. We gathered them in two ways. When the crop was exceedingly large, the ground under the trees would be practically covered with nuts, and these could be swept into piles with a branch of sagebrush, then scooped into a container with the hands. Shaking and winnowing removed any trash. In poorer years the pack rats would gather all the nuts as they fell and store them in their great nests built of pieces of wood, bark, pine cones, cactus, or anything else they could find and carry away. I once found in one of those nests several unexploded sticks of dynamite that the rats had stolen from a local miner. They stored the piñon nuts near the center of their untidy nests, surrounded by shredded cedar bark and protected by spiny cactus needles, but we occasionally raided their hoard.

I still consider these little pine seeds about the finest nuts in existence, and enjoy them either raw or roasted. The newcomer always complains about the tediousness of shelling them, but with long practice one develops a skill that reduces this labor miraculously. The shells are very thin and easily cracked with the teeth, and the piñon has a higher ratio of edible nut to shell than any other nut I know. My father used to hire Indian laborers, and they would often bring no lunch except a bag of piñon nuts. At noon they would sit in the shade and feed these nuts into one corner of their mouths and the empty shells would dribble out the other corner. The whole process of shelling, mastication, and swallowing, went on simultaneously inside their mouths, with never a chewed shell or a wasted piece of edible nut, and in half an hour they had made a good meal. It takes years of practice to acquire this skill, but I have known white boys in New Mexico who could eat piñon nuts in this manner as well as any Indian.

Besides this obvious use as raw or roasted nuts, piñons are also excellent in many kinds of cooking. They make wonderful candies and cookies; simply substitute piñons for whatever nut the recipe calls for. The best turkey stuffing I ever ate had piñon nuts substituted for half the bread crumbs called for in the recipe. These nuts are easily ground in an ordinary food chopper; and the ground nuts cooked as a gruel make one of the best breakfast cereals that nature is capable of producing. When the fine-ground nuts are mixed half-and-half with pancake flour, they make some of the most delicious griddle cakes you ever tasted. Try some of these desert delicacies on your next trip out West.

ARBORVITAE: THE TREE OF LIFE
(*Thuja occidentalis*)

The husky loggers and lumbermen of the north woods during the last century often drank arborvitae tea, partly because they liked it and partly because they thought it gave them strength and prevented illness. They had a song that contained the words:

> A quart of arborvitae
> To make him strong and mighty,

and thought that anyone who drank this aromatic tea regularly would always be free of rheumatism. After trying this tea in several strengths, with and without sugar and milk, I've decided I would almost prefer rheumatism. It is hard to believe that even those tough old loggers drank this tea for pleasure. It has a balsamatic, pungent odor and a taste somewhere between those of camphor and turpentine, with a peculiarly nauseating bitter that is all its own. Maybe one could acquire a taste for it, but, so far, the oftener I drink it the less I like it. If I were suffering from any of the complaints for which arborvitae is said to be the remedy, I might change my mind.

This handsome evergreen member of the pine family is a native of Northeastern United States and adjacent Canada, but it has become so popular as an ornamental that nurserymen have spread it over the land. Today, the easiest place to find arborvitae is not in the north woods but on development lawns, and in parks, cemeteries, and around college campuses. Be very careful about snitching a few leaves from such places to use in home remedies, and I don't mean just be careful not to get caught. Such domesticated arborvitae is sometimes sprayed to control bagworms, and the tea is bad enough at best without adding poisonous insecticide to the brew.

Left to itself, this highly decorative evergreen grows into an even conical shape, twenty to forty feet high, but it can be pruned into any shape, and often is. The dense foliage is made up of flattened leaf sprays of peculiar form. The tender new growth at the tips is used without drying in home remedies. If you don't have an arborvitae growing on your lawn some nearby friend will, and you can probably make arrangements to pick a few sprigs from his tree. If your taste is anything like mine you won't require very much of it.

A strong tea is made by pouring a cup of boiling water over a teaspoonful of the chopped foliage and letting it infuse for about ten minutes. I'm sure that this tea must confer many medicinal benefits, for few other herbal concoctions have so medicinal a taste. It contains several active ingredients and its properties are listed as stimulant, aromatic, astringent, diuretic, and, doubtfully, as an aid in stimulating the menses. It has been used in the past in the treatment of rheumatism, fever, coughs, and delayed menstruation. In my experiments, a cup a day seemed perfectly harmless beyond its unpleasant taste, but this tea should be taken in moderation, a limitation that I find no hardship whatsoever. It is doubtful if anyone ever should "take a quart of arborvitae." Maybe a husky lumberjack who had been drinking it for years could do it, but if you tried it at the first attempt, instead of making you strong and mighty it would probably make you sick. Overdoses have been reported to cause bloating and flatulence and very large overdoses have even caused spasms and convulsions. I can think of few home remedies that I am less tempted to take than an overdose of arborvitae tea.

Despite all I've said against it this may very well be the most active and beneficial herb mentioned in this book. It stimulates both the heart and respiration, and its diuretic action, by increasing the flow of urine, may help the body to rid itself of toxins. A great many people have long believed that arborvitae tea is the best preventive and cure of rheumatism pains that nature provides, and people threatened by, or suffering from, this malady may find this a real tree of life.

20. Stalking the Slippery Elm:

SLIPPERY ELM, RED ELM, OR SWEET ELM

(Ulmus fulva)

I ONCE happened on a television show that was poking fun at health-food restaurants. A man who had never been in such a place before was looking nervously at a menu that listed such items as alfalfa sprout salad, soybean steak, and boiled comfrey. With disgust, he turned to the waiter and said, "Bring me a filet of elm tree." The waiter very calmly replied, "I'm sorry, sir, elm has been out of season for more than a month." In order to make this exchange seem utterly ridiculous, the writer of this script no doubt chose the elm tree as the most obviously inedible plant he could think of. I suspect that the writer would be surprised, however, to learn that his "filet of elm" is not only edible, but very palatable when properly prepared, and furthermore it has long been considered a fine food for infants and invalids, giving wholesome nourishment when the stomach refuses to retain any other food.

The edible elm is the slippery elm, a much smaller tree than the lordly American elm so common as a shade tree. Slippery elm grows in low places and along streams from Quebec to North Dakota and south to Florida and Texas. The outer bark is very rough and deeply furrowed, of a reddish-brown color. The leaves resemble those of the American elm but are larger, hairy underneath, and rough on top, with unevenly toothed margins. The leaf buds in early spring are covered with a yellowish wool. The edible and medicinal part of slippery elm is the white or pinkish inner bark peeled from the trunk or larger limbs. This mucilaginous bark not only is prepared as food, but is an important ingredient in many home remedies, and it is also an official botanical drug in the *National Formulary* and the *U.S. Dispensatory*.

My maternal grandmother would have considered any housewife very remiss who did not keep a supply of slippery-elm bark on hand. "Filet of elm" would never have been out of season in her house. Each spring when the buds were swelling and the sap was running, she would send my uncles out to gather the year's supply of slippery elm, for at that time the bark peels easily from the tree, and the juicy inner bark is easier to detach from the outer, brown bark. They brought this inner bark back home in one- to two-foot strips an inch or so wide and about a quarter-inch in thickness. When spread on papers in an attic room until thoroughly dried, it shrank to no more than an eighth to a sixteenth of an inch in thickness. My grandmother used this dried bark throughout the year in many kinds of foods and home remedies.

Unlike many of the herbs discussed in this book, slippery-elm bark may not be easily available to the hiker or vacationer. One can hardly drive out in the country and start peeling the first slippery-elm tree one can find. However, if you know someone who owns a place in the country, you can usually get permission to peel some of this bark, for the slippery elm is not otherwise a very valuable, nor even a very beautiful tree. Many farmers would be glad to be rid of a few slippery-elm trees.

A few years ago one could buy both the whole dried bark and powdered slippery elm in any drugstore, but recently when I tried to buy some I discovered that it is getting hard to find. A druggist told me that the dried inner bark had been taken off the market because it had been found that some women were using it in a mechanical way to induce abortions. This would be an exceedingly dangerous procedure, not to mention the moral issue involved. It is still permissible to sell the powdered bark, but the demand for it is falling off as people forget how to use it, and it is gradually disappearing from the market. This seems a shame, for it is a pleasant and effective home remedy for many minor complaints and perfectly harmless and safe to use.

Medical books list the properties of slippery elm as demulcent, emollient, expectorant, diuretic, soothing, and nutritive. A few mention it as a mild laxative, but its efficacy in this area is due not to its cathartic drug content, but solely to its lubricative, soothing qualities that enable hard stools to pass comfortably. The most important constituents of this bark are edible mucilage and starch. It is also rich in calcium. It has a soothing, healing effect on all tissues with which it comes in contact, and in addition it is very nutritious when taken internally.

Nearly all slippery-elm recipes use the powdered bark, but in no book could I find directions for powdering it. A few books even said, "powder the bark," which sounds very easy if you say it very fast. I turned again to my trusty blender. I hate to keep mentioning this machine in every chapter, but it has proved to be the handiest appliance in my kitchen, and I have come to the conclusion that anyone messing around with wild foods and healing herbs without having a blender available is wasting his time. Before I could grind it in the blender I had to subject the dried bark to a super-drying to make it more brittle and friable. This was done by laying the dried bark on the rack of a low oven and propping the oven door slightly open so moisture could escape. When a piece of the bark became so brittle that it would snap easily in two when bent, I judged it done.

This extra-dry bark was cut in small pieces, across the grain, then fed into the blender dry, while it was running at high speed. I found it best to grind about one cupful at a time, then empty out the powder before proceeding. The ground bark was put through a very fine sieve, which left me with two products, a very fine, yellowish powder and the coarser material that wouldn't pass through the sieve. Of course I could have sifted after each grind and added the coarse material to the next batch had I wanted all of it powdered, but the coarser material is better for some purposes.

The early settlers learned from the Indians to use slippery elm, and it became one of the most important home remedies in early America. Nearly every writer on herbs of that period mentions the recipe for a medicine that they all, very sensibly, called "slippery-elm food," showing that even in those dim, prescientific days they recognized that the chief value of slippery elm was its nutritive qualities.

To make this simple medicine, simply stir 1 heaping teaspoonful of the fine-powdered bark into enough cold water to make a thin paste, then quickly stir this into 1 pint of boiling water. It can be flavored with a little cinnamon or nutmeg if desired, and can be taken hot or cold. The illnesses for which this slippery-elm drink were given are almost legion. One herbal says,

"Taken unsweetened three times a day, Elm Food gives excellent results in gastritis, gastric catarrh, mucous colitis, and enteritis, being tolerated by the stomach when all other foods fail, and is of great value in bronchitis, bleeding from the lungs and consumption (being most healing to the lungs), soothing a cough and building up and preventing wasting."

As if that weren't enough for one simple home remedy to do, another book says, "It is very good for coughs, colds, influenza, pleurisy, quinsy, dysentery, and painful urination." Still another reference says that a glass of slippery-elm food, taken lukewarm just before going to bed, will induce sleep.

I have tried this slippery-elm food and it wasn't hard to take, but is altogether too much like medicine to please me. As usual, I started experimenting with it. I wondered what would happen if I mixed two excellent demulcents together, so I ground some Irish moss in my blender and mixed it half-and-half with the slippery-elm powder. I then heated a pint of milk in the top of a double boiler and when it was scalding hot, I stirred 2 teaspoonfuls of the mixture into enough cold water to make a paste, then stirred it into the hot milk. I cooked and stirred for about 10 minutes, then strained it through a cloth strainer, sweetened it to taste with honey, and added a dusting of nutmeg for flavor. This was good, and no doubt healing, as a hot drink, going down very smoothly and pleasantly, and when I poured some into a dessert dish and chilled it in the refrigerator, it became a firm junket that was a joy to eat. Here was a medicine to my liking. This was "filet of elm" *deluxe*.

Some herbalists say that the best way to treat colds with slippery elm is to make a stronger drink by pouring a pint of boiling water over 1 ounce of the coarser bark that wouldn't pass through the sieve and allowing it to steep until cool, then adding the juice of ½ lemon and enough honey to sweeten to taste. Here is another medicine I can take, sick or well. This same elm lemonade is highly recommended for feverish patients; allow them to drink all they will take, for this drink will quench their thirst and help relieve their illness by giving them strengthening, easily digested food at the same time.

When I put in long hours writing and pacing my study floor, I am apt to use altogether too much of an American Indian ceremonial herb with the botanical name *Nicotiana Tabacum*, which is rolled into little white cylinders commonly called "cigarettes." Slippery elm has furnished me with a product that not only helps me to cut down on this excessive smoking, but even corrects some of its deleterious effects. I simply put some fine-powdered slippery elm in a bowl, make a little nest in it, pour in a little honey, and carefully work the powder into the honey until it is stiff dough that I can place on a board and cut into small squares. These squares are again rolled in slippery elm, then stored in the refrigerator. They make very effective lozenges, soothing my throat, dispelling my hoarseness, and allaying my cough, and I find that sucking on these lozenges satisfies my infantile oral cravings so that I am not constantly taking another cigarette that I don't really want.

Slippery-elm bark is also highly recommended as a poultice to soothe and help heal inflamed surfaces, wounds, burns, scalds, bruises, and ulcers. These poultices can be used hot or cold, and for this purpose the coarse powder is usually better than the fine. Just work the powder into a paste with hot or cold water, spread it on a bandage, and apply to the affected part. In the chapter on mallows, I have explained how to combine slippery elm with mallows in a poultice, but slippery elm will also combine with many other herb poultices and ointments, adding its soothing demulcent powers to the medicinal benefits of the other herbs.

The Indians formerly ate fresh slippery-elm bark boiled with buffalo meat, and in times of famine both the Indians and the early settlers sometimes subsisted on boiled slippery-elm bark alone. When boiled a long time, this bark reduces to a gelatinous mass from which the fibers are easily removed; the remaining mass is very nourishing and palatable enough so that it would be appreciated by anyone who was really hungry. Even the raw bark is edible and would sustain life in emergencies. I have known many small boys who thoroughly enjoyed chewing on slippery-elm bark in the early spring when it was easy to peel from the tree. The Indians also added slippery-elm bark to the animal fats they rendered for cooking grease, claiming this gave the fat a much better flavor and kept it from becoming rancid. An old farmer once told me that when lard from fall-butchered hogs began to taste rancid in the spring it could be restored to perfect sweetness by melting the whole supply in a large kettle and frying some fresh slippery-elm bark in it. He didn't say how much to use, and I have never had occasion to use this bit of information.

One final use for slippery elm—as I was filleting a mess of fish I had just caught, I wondered how the powdered bark would work as a breading material. I put 2 heaping tablespoons of the fine powder in a paper bag, added ½ teaspoon of salt, ½ teaspoon of monosodium glutamate, and a good dusting of fish garni (a mixture of spices to flavor seafoods). Then I dropped in the fillets, shook them until they were evenly coated and fried them. This Slippery-Elm Breading didn't come off as the fish fried, as do so many coatings. The fish browned very nicely, and those who ate them pronounced them delicious. Slippery elm has too many good uses for us to allow it to become obsolete.

21. The Common Stinging Nettle
(Urtica dioica)

A SURPRISING feature of herbal research is that it is seldom the rare, exotic, and beautiful plant that proves the most interesting; more often it is some common, familiar, and despised weed that is discovered to have undreamed-of virtues. The common nettle is a good illustration. Nearly everyone who has ever run barefoot as a child knows and hates this plant, but it is only a stinging acquaintance. Nettles are common along roadsides, in waste places, and on vacant lots where barefoot children like to play, and when contacted by a bare ankle it causes a painful smarting followed by a red rash. I was recently picking nettles on a nearby farm, and the puzzled farmer wondered aloud why anyone would want to gather "them damn weeds." I started to explain some of the uses of this wonder plant, but he interrupted and said, "All I want to know about nettles is how to get rid of them." This is the attitude that most people have toward this herb.

And yet, this detested weed is one of the finest and most nutritious foods in the whole plant kingdom, a far better vegetable than many of those this same farmer's wife laboriously raises in her kitchen garden. Unlike many health foods, nettle greens are really good, as well as being good for you. People in many parts of the world regularly gather and cook nettle greens, not because they are healthful, but merely because they like them. However, in addition to their good taste, they are rich in vitamins A and C, amazingly high in protein,

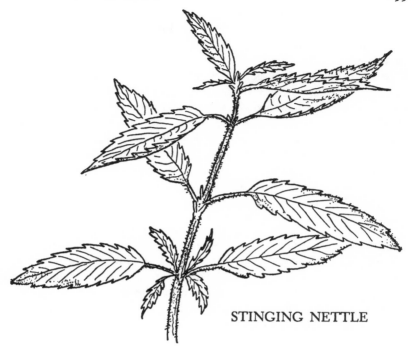

STINGING NETTLE

filled with chlorophyll, and probably exceedingly rich in many of the essential trace minerals.

No grazing animal will eat a live nettle, but when nettles are mowed and dried, all kinds of livestock eat them avidly and thrive on them. Horses get shinier coats and improve in health when fed dried nettles. Cows give more and richer milk when fed on nettle hay. Hens lay more eggs when powdered nettle leaves are added to their mash, and these eggs actually have a higher food value. Turkeys fatten and chicks grow faster when this nutritious food is added to their rations. Powdered dried nettle leaves are actually as rich in protein as cotton-seed meal.

Even the manure from nettle-fed animals is improved, and makes better fertilizer than that from animals not receiving this rich feed. Nettles furnish one of the most valuable of all plant substances to use as a mulch in your garden, or to add to your compost pile. Having approximately seven percent nitrogen, figured on a dry-weight basis, this plant is richer in this essential plant nutrient than many commercial fertilizers. Where nettles grow luxuriantly, there is rich, fertile soil. The British say the best place to locate a new orchard is where nettles like to grow.

All this would seem enough to ask of one common weed, but in addition to these virtues, nettles have also long been used in home remedies and herbal medicines to treat mankind's ills. Any efficacy the nettle may have in this area is probably due to its high content of vitamins and minerals, for I hold to the theory that far more sickness is prevented or cured by proper feeding than by drugging. A lively soft drink can be made of nettles that is reputed to cure the aches and pains of the aged, but it also makes a pleasant beverage for people of all ages.

The stalks of mature nettles yield a valuable textile fiber when processed like flax, and in Scotland, where nettle-linen was formerly made, many people maintain that it is more beautiful and more durable than linen made of flax. Even the sting of the nettle has been thought to be beneficial. Urtication, stinging the flesh with nettles, was an old herbalists' remedy for chronic rheumatism. This wasn't quite the unreasonable superstition that it sounds. Doctors still use counterirritants in treating rheumatic pains, and nettles are certainly efficient counterirritants. Beyond that function, urtication also gave thousands of tiny injections of formic acid, which may have had a positive curative effect. The intuitive and empirical knowledge of those wise in the ways of herbs has often anticipated the findings of scientific medicine by hundreds of years.

Although America has some native nettles that are edible, the common nettle, *Urtica dioica*, was originally a European plant. It was early introduced into this country, quickly became naturalized, and is now found wherever conditions are suitable for its growth. It is usually seen as a small plant, one to two feet high, but in rich stream valleys it may reach a height of six to eight feet. The leaves are opposite, heart-shaped, finely toothed on the margins, and tapering to points. The small green flowers are borne on branched clusters that spring from the axils of the leaves. The whole plant is downy and also covered with stiff stinging hairs. Each sting is really an exceedingly sharp, hollow spine, and arises from a slightly swollen base. This swelling contains the venom that is released through the hollow, polished spine whenever the plant is brushed. The venom is partly formic acid, which accounts for its sharp sting, for it is closely related to the sting of a bee.

When I was a child, we removed the sting of nettles on our skins by rubbing any area affected with the juicy leaves of dock (*Rumex crispus*), which brought almost magical relief. There is a widely held belief that wherever nettles grow, dock will be found growing nearby. Over the years I have formed the habit of looking around for dock whenever I find nettles growing, and I have never failed to find it in reasonably close proximity. However, the converse is not true; dock often grows where there are no nettles. When I was young and innocent, I accepted this arrangement without wonder, considering it the highly sensible arrangement of a beneficent Providence. One didn't just carelessly rub the sting with dock leaves. There was a ritual to it. First a handful of dock leaves were rolled into a ball and squeezed as hard as possible in the hand; then the juice was rubbed onto the affected part while one recited,

> "Nettle in, dock out,
> Dock rub nettle out."

This had to be intoned in just the right key. I must have gotten the charm letter-perfect, for I do not remember the remedy ever failing.

Eating nettles is not at all the unpleasant experience you might expect it to be, for this plant, when gathered at the right stage and properly prepared, is a very palatable vegetable. It is said that a good French cook can make seven delicious dishes of nettle tops. You can do as well, once the general principles of nettle-cookery are known.

Like asparagus, peas, and many other vegetables, nettles must be gathered at just the right stage to be good. The common nettle has perennial underground rhizomes, and from these the tender shoots spring up as soon as the weather is warm. It is only these first nettles, gathered when less than a foot high, that are good to eat. Later in the year, gritty particles called "cystoliths" are deposited in the leaves, making them unpalatable. When nettles are cut down, a new crop springs from the base of the cut plants. I thought surely these newly grown plants would be good, but when I tried some in midsummer they were gritty and gruesome.

Take only the tender tops of young, first-growth nettles, before they begin to bloom. Wear leather or plastic-coated work gloves while gathering nettles, for even these young plants can sting fiercely. Wash the greens by stirring them in water with a long-handled spoon, then use a pair of kitchen tongs to put them directly into a large saucepan with a tight cover. The moisture that clings to the leaves will furnish ample cooking water. Cover and cook gently for twenty minutes; drain, *but save that juice.*

You can chop the greens right in the cooking pot by using a pair of kitchen shears. Season the vegetable with butter and salt to taste, and it is ready to serve. A more wholesome vegetable never came to the table. Formerly this dish not only was considered a palatable, filling, and wholesome food but was also believed to be a powerful medicine, reputed to be useful in treating such diverse diseases as bronchitis, asthma, gout, consumption, diabetes, ague, and even "the stings and bites of venomous creatures and mad dogs," and as an antidote for poisoning by hemlock, henbane, and nightshade. Because of its high vitamin C content, it actually will cure scurvy and other vitamin C deficiency diseases; it was used for this purpose by the herbalists hundreds of years before the term *vitamin* was coined. Its high vitamin A content will help to brighten the eyes, improve night vision, and add gloss to the hair, if their absence is caused by lack of vitamin A.

Cooking completely destroys the nettles' stinging properties, and actually converts the venom into wholesome food.

The information about cooked nettles that moderns will probably find most interesting is that throughout the herbal literature this herb is recommended as being "very efficacious in reducing corpulency." What a wonderful herb! If even half the claims made for nettles are true, and they seem to have truth in them, this one plant can satisfy our hunger, mend our health, delight our taste buds, relieve us of excess poundage, and at the same time give us that virtuous feeling that always seems to envelop any person who is faithfully following a reducing diet.

If you happen not to be wild about plain cooked nettles, don't despair of getting all those benefits, for this is a versatile vegetable that can be prepared in many ways. Try Creamed Nettles: mix the cooked and chopped greens, 2 cupfuls, with a small can of cream of mushroom soup and ½ cup of light cream for a superior creamed vegetable, wonderful over toast. To vary this dish use cream of celery, or some of the new cheese soups, instead of mushroom soup. Another good way to serve nettles is as Puree of Nettles. Rub the cooked nettles, juice and all, through a sieve; return this puree to the heat, add 2 tablespoons of butter, salt to taste, and simmer for about 10 minutes. Remove from the heat, stir in a few tablespoons of light cream, sprinkle with freshly ground black pepper, and serve immediately.

An old English recipe is Nettle Pudding, which is not a dessert, but a hearty main dish that was praised by Pepys in his famous diary. To 2 cups of cooked and chopped nettle greens add 1 cup chopped leek or onion, 1 cup chopped cabbage or broccoli, 1 cup raw rice, 1 cup ground beef, and ½ cup fine-chopped beef suet. Season with 1 teaspoon salt and a little freshly ground black pepper, mix well, then tie the mixture up in a muslin cloth that has been wrung out in cold water. Drop into boiling water and boil for 1 hour, or hang over boiling water and steam for 3 hours. When you remove the pudding cloth, you will have a round cannonball of a pudding that is delicious when served with a good gravy or melted butter.

I play around with this Nettle Pudding recipe. Sometimes I substitute Chinese cabbage for the broccoli, add a bit of grated green ginger to the mix, and serve it with hot Chinese mustard and soy sauce as a rare find among Oriental dishes. Other times I use a cup of chopped celery, add a minced clove of garlic and a package of dry spaghetti mix, and come up with a delicious Italian dish that has probably never been eaten in Italy. I'll bet you could add some chili powder and oregano and get away with calling it a Mexican dish, or put in some chopped eggplant and curry powder and pass it off as a recipe you discovered in India. You can also substitute nettle greens in any recipe that calls for spinach, chard, turnip greens, or beet tops, but we have already left those French cooks far behind.

Let's return to that juice we drained from the cooked nettles. Just seasoned with a little salt and pepper and a very little vinegar, it makes a tasty soup that is supposed to be very efficacious in removing unwanted pounds. Mixed with a little honey it is said to relieve asthma, allay a cough, and help cure bronchitis. Taken as hot as you can drink it, after exposure, this juice has a reputation of helping to prevent colds. I know it is a nice warming drink on a chilly day, giving a warm glow all over.

This same juice, cooled, is said to be a fine hair tonic. Applied twice a day it is reputed to prevent falling hair, eliminate dandruff, promote a healthy scalp, and help to keep the hair neatly combed.

When one adds as much common table salt to this juice as it will absorb, the mixture acquires the ability to coagulate milk, like rennet. To make a delicious Nettle Junket, heat 1 pint of milk in the top of a double boiler to just lukewarm, then stir in 2 tablespoons of sugar, ½ teaspoon of vanilla, and 1 teaspoon of salted nettle juice, then pour into the glasses or dishes from which it will be eaten, and chill. For variety you can substitute a square of unsweetened chocolate, or any other flavoring or spice that suits your fancy for the vanilla, or serve the junket covered with fresh berries or other fruit.

In some parts of England the country people still make a pleasant summer drink called Nettle Beer. To 4 quarts of freshly picked nettle tops add 2 gallons of water, 2 lemons cut in thin slices, rind and all, and 2 ounces of crushed, dried gingerroot. Boil gently for forty minutes, then strain and stir in 2 cups of brown sugar. When cooled to barely lukewarm, dissolve a cake of yeast in a cup of the liquid and then stir it into the brew. Bottle immediately and cap tightly, and in a few days it is ready to drink. It should be refrigerated until ice-cold before opening, for this is a lively drink and will foam wildly if opened while warm. It is considered a good beverage for old people, relieving their gouty and rheumatic pains, but the whole family will enjoy it, and since it has no detectable alcoholic content it can be given to children and members of Alcoholics Anonymous.

Probably no other wild plant so perfectly demonstrates the change of attitude one experiences toward weeds when their virtues become known. To one who knows the nettle only by its sting, it is a weed to be avoided and detested, but once you know how many ways it can serve you, although you will still respect its defense mechanism, you will also experience a glow of satisfaction every time you see a patch of stinging nettles.

22. Marsh-Marigold or American Cowslip

(*Caltha palustris*)

ALTHOUGH I call this plant "American cowslip" in the heading, it is not peculiar to America. Exactly the same species grows in England, but it is never called "cowslip" there. In England the term "cowslip" means *Primula veris*, a wild flower related to the primrose and pimpernel, not only differing from our cowslip in genus and species, but belonging to an entirely different family of plants. The same name being applied to two widely different plants has caused confusion. A very recent American book on wild foods slips on its own cowslips. It tells how to preserve uncooked cowslip blossoms in sugar, taking the recipe from an old English source, apparently not realizing that these directions were for an altogether different flower. Obviously the author did not test this recipe before publishing it, for marsh-marigolds preserved in this manner would be extremely acrid and pungent. Had the author consumed much of this confection he would never have been guilty of recommending this untried recipe, for the uncooked marsh-marigold contains a poisonous glucoside, which is expelled by boiling.

If using the term "cowslip" for this plant leads to confusion, its alternate common name, marsh-marigold, is little better, for neither is it related to the marigold. The English have about two dozen common names for the plant we call cowslip, but most of them are unknown on this side of the Atlantic. An ideal common name for this plant would be "marsh buttercup," for it is closely related to the

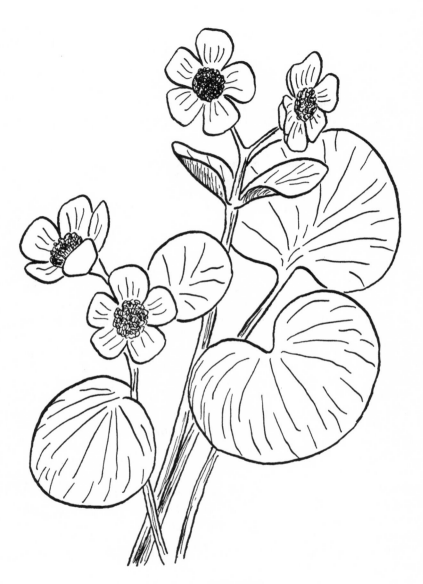

MARSH-MARIGOLD

common buttercups, and the flower, though much larger, more closely resembles a buttercup than it does either the European cowslip or the marigold. However, language exists to help us communicate, and if I began calling it "marsh buttercup" no one would know the plant I meant. I guess I'll have to continue to call it *cowslip* or *marsh-marigold*, even if I have to explain that I am not talking about a real cowslip or a real marigold at all.

In America the marsh-marigold is a common wildflower in swamps, marshy places, sluggish streams, and wet meadows, from Newfoundland to South Carolina and west to Nebraska. It has hollow, branching stems, 12 to 18 inches tall. The basal leaves are on long, fleshy leafstalks, while the upper leaves are almost stalkless. The leaf-blades are three to six inches across, heart-shaped or kidney-shaped, with margins that may be smooth or wavy, or sometimes have rounded teeth. The five-petaled flowers appear in April or May, and they are bright yellow, about an inch and a half across, and resemble giant buttercups.

As a medicinal herb the marsh-marigold has been used in treating warts, fits, dropsy, and anemia. It is also said to have expectorant and pectoral properties, making it a valuable ingredient in cough syrups, but I have so many herbal cough syrups around the house now that I refuse to make another one. To all these virtues I would like to add that it is nutritious, for Boiled Cowslip Greens are the favorite pot-herb of many foragers, and there is no doubt that this is an exceedingly wholesome vegetable when properly prepared. For centuries rains have been leaching essential mineral salts from higher, well-drained lands and depositing them in the swamps and marshes. Food plants raised on the high, leached-out soils are apt to be deficient in minerals and vitamins. It is the edible marsh plants that can give us our full quota of these essential nutrients to keep us in glowing health. The dark-green leaves of the marsh-marigold, with their rich underlying yellow pigment, show that we can expect high yields of vitamins C and A when this plant is explored for its nutritional benefits. The use of marsh-marigold in treating anemia was a reasonable one, for this deep-green plant of the low, mineral-rich marshes is undoubtedly rich in iron, a nutrient necessary for building healthy red blood.

Uncooked marsh-marigold is very acrid and pungent, and its only medicinal use in this raw state that I know is as a home remedy for warts. A drop of the caustic juice is squeezed from the leaf or stem onto the wart every day until is disappears. Warts, especially on children's hands, come and go with no apparent rhyme or reason, but maybe this pungent juice does hurry their going. There are literally dozens of wart cures in the old herbal literature. It is very hard to determine when a wart has been cured by any treatment, for apparently warts are sometimes cured by faith alone. I read an article by a reputable doctor who said that whenever he noticed a wart on one of his patients, he made a great to-do over treating it with some completely inert substance and assured the patient that it would soon be gone, and usually it was. There is a theory that warts are due to a shortage of vitamin A in the diet, and if this is true, warts could be prevented or cured by eating cowslip greens for their carotene content.

Marsh-marigold was formerly used in the treatment of "fits"—a term used for some of the convulsive disorders we now lump together under the term *epilepsy*. One book says that an infusion of the flowers was "successfully used in various kinds of fits, both of children and adults." Dr. Withering, the famous English physician of the 18th century, who lifted *digitalis* from an old wives' herbal remedy to an important medicine that is still highly respected by the medical profession, also experimented with marsh-marigold. He suggests a strange use for this plant:

"It would appear that medicinal properties may be evolved in the gaseous exhalations of plants and flowers, for on a large quantity of the flowers of Meadow Routs [one of the many English common names of the marsh-marigold] being put into the bedroom of a girl who had been subject to fits, the fits ceased."

If you would like to do something nice for someone who suffers from epilepsy, "Say it with flowers."

I have not attempted to make any medicines from marsh-marigolds, for on studying its uses I concluded that I could get all its medicinal benefits, real or fancied, by eating Cowslip Greens. Besides, they are good. Only a vandal would pull up the plants while gathering these greens. Put on some hip boots and prepare to spend a little time among these beautiful flowers. Prime leaves can be cut from their long petioles with a pair of shears or a penknife without injuring the plant. Wash the leaves, then cover them with boiling water. Bring this water back to a boil, and immediately drain. Add more boiling water and repeat the process. After two of these hot-water treatments, or even three if you want extra mild greens, cook the leaves in very little water until tender, chop, and season with butter, salt, and a little cider vinegar.

Some health-food enthusiasts will object that these hot-water treatments will leach out all the vitamins and minerals, but this is not entirely true. These leaves are subjected to no more hot water than are vegetables being prepared for the freezer, and experiments indicate that this blanching not only does not destroy many vitamins, but actually helps to prevent those left from deteriorating. Besides, untreated cowslips would be too acrid and pungent to eat, and they might even poison you.

Most people appreciate the slight pungency of Cowslip Greens, but for those who demand an absolute absence of bite from their vegetables these greens can be creamed, making them very mild and bland but retaining some of their characteristic good flavor. A good method of preparing them is to combine 2 cups of the cooked, chopped greens, prepared as directed above, with ½ cup of rich milk, and a small can of cream of mushroom soup. Cook and stir until all ingredients are thoroughly mixed and slightly thickened, add salt and pepper to taste, and serve.

The unopened flower buds of marsh-marigold make an excellent Marsh-Marigold Condiment-Pickle that can be used like capers. For this purpose gather only the still-tightly-closed buds and give them the same kind of double hot-water treatment recommended for the leaves. Drain well and put the buds in a pint jar. In a saucepan combine 1 cup of vinegar, ½ cup of water, ¼ cup of sugar, a tablespoon of salt, a teaspoon of mustard seed, and a teaspoon of celery seed, and boil for 10 minutes. Pour this over the buds boiling hot, and seal the jar with a sterilized, domed two-piece lid. These should not be opened for at least a month, and then use only the buds, discarding the liquid.

To make a delicious Cowslip Sauce, melt 1 tablespoon of butter in a saucepan, then stir in 2 tablespoons of flour until it is smooth. Add 1 small can of bouillon, and cook and stir until it just comes to a boil. Add ½ cup of well-drained pickled cowslip buds, and it is ready to serve. More luxurious than a mushroom sauce.

Some may think that I am doing the marsh-marigold a disservice by pointing out its value as a food plant, but the conscientious forager protects his source of supply by never destroying the plant that is feeding him. The only marsh-marigolds I ever pulled are those I transplant to some new spot suitable for their growth, and I have considerably increased my foraging area in this way. The chief danger to the marsh-marigold is not from those who would use a few of its leaves and flower buds for food, but from those who think that every marsh or swamp should be drained or filled, in the name of reclamation. I will admit that such projects are sometimes necessary, but if everyone who contemplated filling or draining a marsh or swamp would first take the time to become thoroughly acquainted with all the lifeforms that would perish in such an operation, I feel sure that we would shortly consider far fewer of them necessary. Now we change the earth in almost total ignorance of the names, natures, and virtues of the plants and animals we are destroying with our earth-moving machinery, and to add insult to injury, we call our destruction "conservation" or "reclamation." The Devil laughs.

23. Goldthread, Canker-root, or Mouthroot

(Coptis groenlandica)

THIS IS a small herb, not over five inches high, with three-part evergreen leaves resembling those of the strawberry. It is common over New England and eastern Canada, growing in sphagnum bogs and swamps, and it comes south to Maryland in the mountains and has been reported from as far west as Iowa. In the southern part of its range it is often found in rich, damp woods. In late spring or early summer the plant bears a white, star-shaped flower about one inch across. For more certain identification, pull up the plant and examine the roots. Goldthread has branching, matted, threadlike roots that are a bright golden color. These bright-yellow roots are the medicinal part of the herb.

Goldthread roots furnish one of the purest, clearest, cleanest-tasting bitters to be found in all nature, with no nausating properties and not a hint of astringency. There is no odor whatever. The herb is still in reasonably constant demand in this country. A closely related species of *Coptis* (its botanical name) is highly regarded as a medicine in India and China. It is used as a bitter tonic to stimulate the appetite and is thought to be especially valuable during convalescence, when nourishing food is needed and the appetite is inclined to be dull. It is also used as a mouthwash to cure thrush and all kinds of mouth sores.

To prepare the medicine, steep 2 teaspoons of the fine-chopped root in 1 pint of boiling water for 20 minutes, then strain. Take a

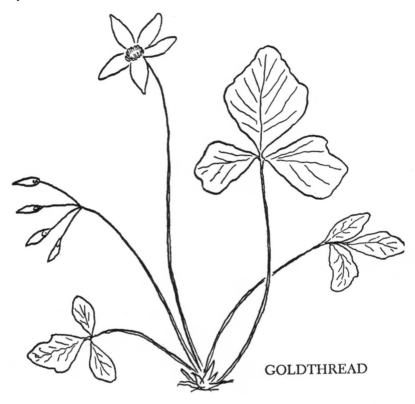

GOLDTHREAD

tablespoon of the infusion half an hour before meals as an appetite stimulant, and take as much as 6 tablespoons a day as a mouthwash for sores in the mouth.

Of what use is this bitter herb to a perfectly well man? I believe it can help keep him well and help him to enjoy other food. As I have indicated, a taste for bitters must be acquired, but this does not deprecate bitters in any way. Have you ever noticed how soon we tire of flavors that seem delicious at the first taste? The sweet, the mild, and the bland soon pall, but the bolder, more rugged flavors for which we must acquire a liking are much more durable. Our grandfathers knew how to appreciate bitters, but the practice of taking bitters before or with meals is much older than that. The ancient Greek and Roman gourmets considered bitters necessary to the enjoyment of food. Some say that plant breeders, food refiners, and excellent cooks have so improved our food that bitters are no longer necessary for its enjoyment, but I doubt that this is the reason for the modern neglect of this taste. I find much modern food exceedingly tasteless. Others say that the overfed and overweight generation is much more interested in things that will inhibit the appetite than in those things that will stimulate it, but isn't it just these mild, bland, sweet, and starchy foods, that have so little taste one can almost eat them without knowing it, that are putting on all these excess pounds? When food has a strong, pronounced flavor it is impossible to eat it in this absentminded manner. When I eat foods that have authoritative, attention-getting flavors, I find that I am satisfied with much less. In my opinion, the present neglect of bitters is due only to fashion. There are fashions in food and drink, just as there are fashions in dress, coiffures, and make-up, and these styles change, often in a cyclic, repetitive fashion. I predict that bitters are about to make a grand comeback. They already have, as far as I'm concerned.

Despite my interest in medicinal herbs I have a strong bias against taking medicine, believing that if people would only eat and drink the right things in the right quantities most medicines would be unnecessary. Naturally I started looking for a more pleasant way of taking goldthread than as a medicine taken from a tablespoon. About this time a woman wrote, asking me to help her devise a good recipe for homemade root beer that would use only natural roots and barks of wild plants that grew in her locality. I sat down and thought of the flavors that I would appreciate in a root beer. There should be a sweet and a sour, but not too much of either. There should be a strong but pleasant aromatic flavor and a good bitter to keep it from tasting weak and characterless. In addition there should be a demulcent to keep it from being too thin and watery and to give it enough smoothness to go pleasantly down the throat.

This woman lived in Massachusetts, near the sea, and being limited to the plants she had mentioned in her letter, I chose sassafras roots as the aromatic, Irish moss as the demulcent, and goldthread as the bitter. Ordinary sugar would furnish the sweet, and the slight fermentation and subsequent carbonation would furnish the acid. I used ½ pound of dried sassafras-root bark and 2 ounces of dried Irish moss tied up together in a cheesecloth bag. This bag was boiled for 30 minutes in 2 gallons of water; then I added another bag containing about 2 ounces of well-washed roots of goldthread, and removed the brew from the heat. After letting it steep until merely lukewarm, I removed the herb bags and added 2 cups sugar and 1 teaspoon of dry, active yeast that had first been dissolved in a little of the liquid.

After standing in a warm room for about 6 hours, it was bubbling nicely, so I bottled it, sealing the bottles with crown caps. When it had been stored in my cellar for a week it cleared up, so I put a bottle of it in the refrigerator for a day, then sampled it. It was lively and foaming, though not holding its "head" as long as commercial root beer. The sassafras had contributed a reddish color and the goldthread a bright yellow so the resulting blend was a pleasing orange-amber. It tasted a little—very little—like commercial root beer. It was stronger in flavor and less sweet, with some bold overtones that were all its own. When drunk before lunch or dinner, it did not depress my appetite or dull my taste buds as spiritous liquors do. A single glass of it sharpens my appetite and seems to make good food taste even better.

Since this beer is bottled as soon as fermentation starts, there are only minute quantities of alcohol formed, so, for all intents and purposes, it can be regarded as a non-alcoholic drink that can be given to children and teetotalers. Indeed, goldthread once had a great reputation as a cure for alcoholism, and a decoction of these bright-yellow roots was reputed to destroy the taste for alcoholic beverages of all kinds. With several other herbs it was part of the once-famous "Gold Cure" for problem drinkers, so maybe you should encourage those who imbibe too freely to try your Goldthread Root Beer.

24. Wild Carrot, Bird's-nest, or Queen Anne's-lace

(*Daucus Carota*)

THE WILD CARROT is not native to America, but since the coming of the white man it has become naturalized everywhere, sometimes growing in solid stands in old fields. It is a biennial, producing the familiar feathery carrot foliage the first year and a stringy, white, slender root. The foliage dies down at the coming of winter, but the root survives. The second year, the root puts out new foliage and a stout, furrowed seedstalk, and all the books I have referred to agree that this seedstalk may grow to a height of two feet. Indeed it may! I can look out my study window and see hundreds of dried wild carrot stalks rising above the snow, a great many of them more than three feet high and some of them standing more than four feet tall.

The second-year wild carrot begins blooming in June and continues to bloom until September, and during this time it is a thing of beauty. The individual blossoms are small, but they are densely clustered together in terminal umbels, or flattened heads, some of them as large as a saucer. These flowering umbels are quite decorative and give the plant its most widely used common name: Queen Anne's-lace. These flowers are milky white, but strangely, if you look closely you will nearly always find one little flower near the center of the flat umbel that is pink, red, or purple. There was formerly a superstition in England that eating these colored flowers would cure epilepsy.

The tiny flowers in the large umbel are followed by an abundant

149

setting of seed, and as the seeds ripen, the umbel begins resembling a cup more than a saucer. The edges turn up and inward, enclosing a hollow space. It is the brown seed head of such peculiar shape that gives this plant its other common name: bird's-nest.

The wild carrot is widespread in many lands now, but it was probably originally a native of the Mediterranean area, and it has a venerable history of use in herbal medicines. The plant is mentioned by Greek writers who lived five hundred years before Christ, and even then domestic varieties had already been developed and were being cultivated for food, and the wild ones had many uses in the ancient *materia medica.*

Probably no other plant so well illustrates what can be done by plant breeding, seed selection, and cultivation as the ordinary carrot. It always amazes me how few people recognize that the rich orange-colored, crisp, and delicious garden carrot and the common old-field weed, Queen Anne's-lace, are exactly the same species, with only varietal differences. Whenever I point out that these two are really the same plant, the first reaction always is, "Did our domestic carrot come from that weed?" Then I have another surprise ready. In America there is a far greater probability that "that weed" came from the domestic carrot!

Garden carrots can sometimes "go wild" in a single generation. In almost every planting of carrots there will be a few atavistic specimens that will produce white, tough, slender little roots that are not worth gathering. If these roots are left in the ground and allowed to seed, the next summer they will be indistinguishable from the wild Queen Anne's-lace, and their seed will produce only wild types.

Good carrots never get a chance to go wild. Even if good carrots are abandoned or overlooked by the human beings who planted them, they will not be overlooked by the rabbits, field mice, chipmunks, and other rodents who know a good carrot when they taste it. These hungry little animals will see to it that a good carrot never gets a chance to set seed. Commercial seed producers must select the very best roots, protect them from the depredations of wild creatures, and raise seed from them the second year in order to preserve our improved garden varieties. To take this process full circle, there is a report that a woman in Maine planted wild carrot seed, cultivated them, selected the best roots, and gradually redomesticated them into a new variety that she described as remarkably sweet.

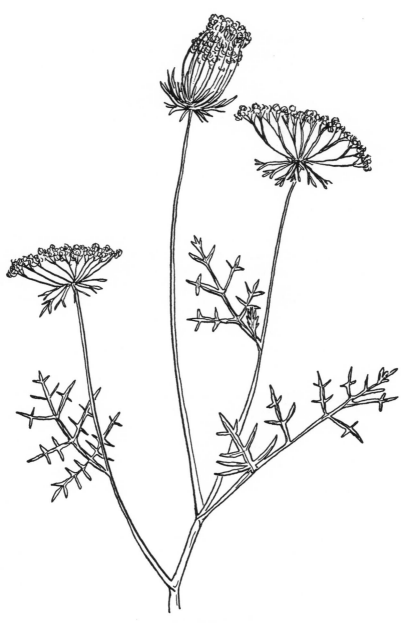

WILD CARROT

There is a curious belief among my Pennsylvania Dutch neighbors that Queen Anne's-lace is poisonous, which probably arose from the fact that livestock dislike its aromatic flavor and mostly refuse to eat it. First-year roots, in the fall, are small, tough, and uninviting, but they continue to grow, very slowly, of course, over the winter, and by spring are often as large as your finger and up to six inches long. These overwintered roots are easily located when they send up the first of their tiny, feathery green leaves, and dug at this time they are perfectly edible. Last spring I followed a neighbor as he plowed a field that had been badly infested with wild carrot and selected the largest and finest roots, and got a good supply for my experiments with very little labor.

These roots are easily identified by anyone with a normal nose, for they have exactly the same smell as garden carrots, although they are white instead of yellow or orange. I washed my wild carrots, scraped them, boiled them in just enough water to cover for about 20 minutes, and they became very tender. These were seasoned with salt and butter, and I ate quite a large plate of them with no ill effects whatever. They were quite good, with a distinctly recognizable carrot flavor. They were not as sweet as garden carrots, and of course they lack the yellow carotene that makes the garden carrot such a healthful vegetable. There was a tough woody core at the center of each one of the wild carrots, but these easily slipped out when the carrot was cooked, and the rest of it was pretty good food. I won't say I preferred them to garden carrots, but they would make an excellent emergency, or survival, food and would be fine to add a carrot flavor and much food value to a camp stew if cultivated carrots were not available.

The roots, the foliage, and the seeds of wild carrots are used in home remedies that come highly recommended by the old herbalists. The feathery first-year foliage is gathered and dried in a warm room, then used to make an infusion, 1 ounce of the herb steeped in 1 pint of boiling water, and taken in wineglassful doses night and morning. This remedy is said to be diuretic, stimulating, and an aid in clearing natural ducts of the body, and is called "an active and valuable remedy in the treatment of dropsy, chronic kidney diseases, and affections of the bladder." It also "is very useful in gravel and stone, and is good against flatulence," and "is considered excellent for lithic acid and a gouty disposition." I'm afraid I know some people who should be given this remedy forcibly. I can only vouch for the fact that it is a warming aromatic drink with a familiar carroty flavor and seems to be harmless in action.

The fleshy roots, boiled until tender, the hard cores removed, and the soft parts mashed and applied warm, are said to make a good poultice for boils, carbuncles, ulcers, and infected skin punctures, helping to allay pain and bring boils and carbuncles to a head.

The best product of the wild carrot is the seeds that are so abundantly produced. These seeds are not difficult to gather. Simply go out in an old field and thresh the loaded seed heads, by hand, directly into a container. You won't need more than a cupful or two unless you are planning to go into the herb business. They are easily cleaned by rubbing between the hands to loosen the chaff and winnowing in a very light breeze. Wild carrot seed, like the seeds of many of its relatives such as celery, dill, anise, and caraway, make an excellent spice or flavoring material. To make this spice, powder the seeds in a blender and put through a fine flour sifter to remove any chaff or large particles. This spice can add a new dimension to soups, stew, boiled meats, or goulash. Add it early, as it requires cooking to bring out its best flavor.

As an herbal medicine the seeds are said to be carminative and stimulating and very useful in flatulence, windy colic, hiccups, dysentery, chronic coughs, calculus or body "stone" complaints, obstruction of the viscera, jaundice, dropsy, and suppressed menstruation. Nearly anyone should be able to pick from such a lengthy list at least one excuse for drinking Carrot Seed Tea. I drink it because I like it. The seeds of wild carrot and anise have much the same properties, and I have discovered that a tea made by combining the seeds of these two closely related plants is more palatable than tea made with either one alone. A pint of boiling water poured over 1 tablespoonful of crushed carrot seeds and 1 tablespoonful of crushed anise seeds makes a warm, fragrant, aromatic tea that I can enjoy. Because of its reputed gas-reducing properties, this spicy tea, served as a demitasse at the end of a rich meal, would not only be an interesting and attention-getting change from the usual after-dinner coffee, but would also be some insurance against your guests developing any distressing aftereffects from your cooking. These seeds are said to be a genuine aid in digesting carbohydrates properly and in preventing flatulence. I think the wild carrot is an herb worth knowing.

25. Ginseng:

MORE PRECIOUS THAN GOLD

(*Panax quinquefolium*)

GINSENG! The very name sings of romance, and this lowly plant
has a more romantic history than any herb I know. Confucius
praised its curative powers more than 2,000 years ago, and it has remained central in the Chinese *materia medica* ever since, and is
added to many of their favorite prescriptions even today. For centuries the Chinese obtained ginseng from Manchuria, Chinese Tur-
kestan, and Korea, but gradually the supply was depleted and prices
rose to fantastic levels. This was the Asiatic species, *Panax schinseng*
—*Panax* from the same root as panacea, a cure-all, and *schinseng*,
from which we took our word, ginseng, being the Chinese name for
the highly-valued medicinal root of this plant.

Schinseng, in Chinese, means man-form, or man-shape, for the
small root of ginseng often divides at the bottom into two leg-shaped
forks, and sometimes has arm-like side roots higher up, resembling a
tiny man in some grotesque posture. Some scholars ascribe the value
placed on this root to the old doctrine of signatures, conjecturing
that ancient medicine men interpreted its man-shape to mean that it
would be a good medicine for man to take. This may have been true
in the dim, primitive past, but the modern, educated Chinese of
Formosa, Macao, Hong Kong, or Singapore still value the root as
highly as did their honorable ancestors, and will pay a higher price
for it than for any other drug on the market.

We speak of something very valuable being worth its weight in
gold, but a perfect, unbroken, particularly human-shaped root of

ginseng, cured to a clear translucency by a secret process known only to Chinese druggists, may bring as much as $300 to $400 *an ounce* in the Orient, and that is roughly ten times the world price of gold. Such a root, encased in fine silk and presented in a little jeweled casket, is considered an appropriate and ingratiating gift for a powerful and revered Chinese patriarch, for ginseng is considered an herbal fountain of youth and is peculiarly the medicine of the old.

Back in the 18th century, some enterprising Yankee in the China trade examined this much-sought-after plant in Asia and realized that a very similar species grew in his native New England. On his next trip to the Orient, he took along several hundred pounds of this American ginseng and returned home a great deal richer than when he left. The great ginseng boom was on.

The American species, *P. quinquefolium*, is a small, unassuming plant, ten to twenty inches high, that grows from Quebec to Manitoba and southward, chiefly in the hill districts, to Alabama and Arkansas. It likes shady ravines or gentle north slopes where the soil is light, well-drained, and rich with leaf mold from hardwood forests. It is a slow grower, taking a full year to get started. In the second year it puts up two leaves, each divided into five pointed leaflets. In the third year it adds another leaf and produces some greenish-yellow flowers that are followed by clusters of red berries containing pea-sized wrinkled seeds. It takes ginseng five to eight years to produce a root of salable size. This root is two to four inches long, cylindrical or spindle-shaped, with prominent circular wrinkles, usually forked and often with two or three side roots above the fork. Very few of these roots are truly man-shaped before some of the extra "arms" and "legs" are trimmed off.

At the time it was discovered that ginseng could be sold at a great profit, New England had already been settled more than a hundred years, and many of her forests were gone. Ginseng had already dwindled from want of shade, leaf mold, and a solitary place in which to grow. The little that was left soon fell prey to greedy collectors, and the source of easy money rapidly dwindled to the vanishing point. However, by this time, Americans were pushing across the Appalachians, and it was discovered that ginseng had a wider range than had been suspected. Few now realize the important role ginseng played in the settlement of these new western lands. It was one of the few commodities valuable enough to transport to eastern markets by the primitive means then available and still show a profit.

In some of the early settlements in Minnesota, ginseng made the difference between success and failure. Many of the first settlers borrowed money to help them establish farms in the wilderness, and a series of natural disasters, including several unusually severe winters, locust plagues, and crop failures, dogged them. Then came the panic and depression of 1857–1858, their loans were called in, and whole neighborhoods were left bankrupt. Just when these pioneers were about ready to give up, traders arrived from the East and acquainted them with the value of this insignificant little plant that grew so abundantly in their cool forests. Whole communities turned to hunting ginseng, and even the neighboring Indian tribes got into the act. Thousands of dollars began pouring into the impoverished settlements, enabling them to survive until they had built their frontier economy up to a self-sustaining level. Of course these backwoodsmen received only a tiny fraction of the price this root would eventually bring when retailed in China to rich old aristocrats, but since they had not formerly known that this plant had any value at all, the price of several dollars per pound they received for the roots seemed fabulous.

The money from ginseng enabled these hardy pioneers to settle permanently in many new areas, but the peak of the ginseng boom was soon passed. Ginseng doesn't grow in huge patches, but is usually solitary. It is such a slow grower that with everyone on the lookout for this valuable plant the supply of full-grown roots was soon exhausted. The demand in China did not lessen, and any ginseng that could be found could still be sold. Although the prices fluctuated wildly during the early years, and have trended steadily upward, the plant became so rare that hunting for it was no longer profitable.

In a few areas, small quantities of wild ginseng are still found and sold every year, even now, but in most communities where this valuable root was formerly an important secondary source of income, the search for it gradually ceased altogether. A new generation grew up that did not even recognize the plant. Fortunately, a few young plants and a few sprouting seeds escaped the earlier depredations, and slowly, almost secretly, ginseng began re-establishing itself in the few suitable habitats left to it. Now it is making a real comeback, and there is probably more wild ginseng in America today than there was fifty years ago.

Early in this century, there was another kind of boom in ginseng, but this one put very few roots on the shelves of Chinese druggists. As the supply of wild ginseng declined, it was only natural to think of raising it under cultivation. Smart promoters began selling plants and advertising that here was the way to make huge fortunes with small plantings of this expensive drug plant. The plant suppliers did very well, but not one in ten of the suckers that were taken in by this skin game ever produced a single salable root of ginseng. This plant requires very special conditions in order to thrive, and these conditions are hard to duplicate under cultivation; too much sun and only slightly unsuitable soil conditions could easily kill a whole plantation. Some of these get-rich-quick growers tried to hurry the plants by adding commercial fertilizer or barnyard manure, only to discover that these materials had killed their young plants. Most, however, merely became impatient at the long time it takes a ginseng root to mature; they lost interest in the project, let their shading sheds fall down, and allowed weeds to crowd out the noncompetitive ginseng.

A few of the entrepreneurs did raise ginseng successfully, but even they found that the profits from this unusual crop fell far short of what the promoters had promised. As a get-rich-quick scheme it was a failure, but when cultivated ginseng was handled with skill, diligence, and attention to detail, it did yield a fair return on initial investment and the time spent raising it.

I know one man who raises ginseng successfully, though he considers it more his hobby than any substantial contributor to his income. When this man was a boy, he was one of the last professional ginseng gatherers in this part of Pennsylvania, so ginseng is a plant of happy memories to him. He told me that he once collected three pounds of wild ginseng in one day, at a time when it was selling for nine dollars a pound. Twenty-seven dollars was more than most boys of that time could make in a month.

Having known wild ginseng all his life, he knew the growing conditions it required, and when he decided to try raising ginseng for fun he knew exactly how to duplicate those conditions. He hauled in forest leaf mold and made deep, rich beds and shaded them with a pole shed supported by durable locust posts, then trained wild frost-

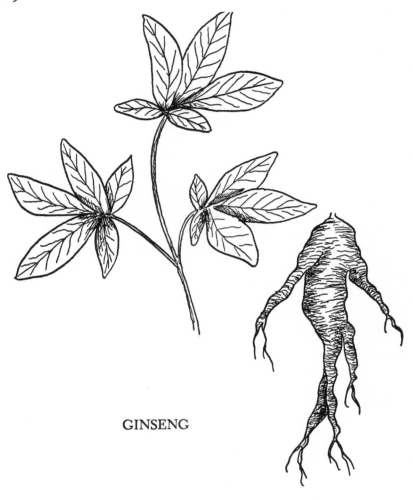

GINSENG

grape vines over the shed to give shade in summer and allow the sun
to peep through in the winter after the grape leaves had fallen. He
kept the beds of young plants free of weeds, mulched them every fall
with a blanket of fallen leaves, gave them another top dressing of
forest leaf mold every spring, and used no other fertilizers. Each
year, for eight wears, he extended his pole shed and prepared and
planted new ginseng beds.

At the end of the first eight years, he harvested the roots from the first bed and replanted it. Now, one section of his plantation is ready for harvest every year, and while it hasn't made him rich, it is one of the best-paying hobbies I ever encountered. His neat ginseng beds under their extensive arbor of grape vines make a popular show-place in the neighborhood, attracting considerable attention. His latest crop commanded a price of more than thirty dollars a pound. He also harvests the little frost-grapes from the shading vines and makes them into a spicy grape wine that helps to while away long winter evenings.

I wonder how much of this expensive drug is still used in Communist China? In 1962, we shipped more than a hundred thousand pounds of ginseng to Hong Kong, and I'm sure some of it found its way across the border. However, the ginseng hunters and growers of America do not have to depend on Communist China for a market. There are many millions of Chinese in Southeast Asia, outside China, many of them wealthy merchants who can afford to indulge in such high-priced medication. These exiled Sons of the Celestial Empire are ready and eager to buy far more ginseng than we produce.

What is so wonderful about ginseng that the Chinese will pay these princely prices for it? Frankly, I don't know. Our own doctors admit that it is a fair stomachic and bitter tonic, and that it acts as a very mild heart and respiration stimulant, but it has long been discarded by most Western pharmacopoeias as worthless. Among the Chinese it is given to the sick to make them well and to the well to keep them from getting sick. It is believed to be a powerful aphrodisiac, especially efficacious in restoring vim, vigor, and the vitality of manhood to old and impotent men. But even more important, the regular use of ginseng is believed to greatly prolong life, and in Chinese families, where the old are honored simply because they are old, it is worth while trying to prolong existence into extreme old age. These reputed powers would easily explain why the root is so highly valued, if they could be proved to exist, but Western scientists maintain that all these Chinese uses of ginseng are utterly without any scientific justification. I wonder ... ?

During the last few years, I have done considerable walking and exploring in Pennsylvania woodlands, and I have always kept my eye out for ginseng. I have collected the grand total of five roots, averaging about an ounce apiece. Even at the prices this root brings, such a quantity could not make much difference in my financial status, so

I decided to enjoy the luxury of using such an expensive product myself. The root should be dug from the ground, not pulled, to prevent breaking the precious little "arms" and "legs." Clean the root with hot water and a small brush, working on it until you have removed the last speck of dirt or stain. Dry it in an airy room.

One of my precious few roots was partly used for tasting purposes, both fresh and dried, and while it wasn't absolutely nauseating, I felt sure the Chinese didn't pay those prices merely to enjoy the taste. It was both bitter and sweet, with aromatic overtones, but no one would call it delicious. The rest of this root, about a half-ounce dried, was shaved fine and covered with a pint of boiling water and allowed to steep until it was cold. I took about an ounce of this decoction every morning until I used it up. The taste wasn't bad, but neither was it anything to brag about. According to the Chinese, such Ginseng Tea will cure consumption and ward off any number of horrible illnesses. I could detect no difference in my health while drinking this infusion, but the feeling of luxurious self-indulgence that came from drinking a beverage that would have cost a Chinese a king's ransom was terrific.

I used two of the roots, totalling 2 ounces dry weight, to make a Ginseng Tincture for which I found the recipe in an old herbal. This called for covering 1 part of powdered ginseng root with 5 parts grain alcohol, so I cut my two little roots into fine pieces, put them in my trusty blender, added 10 ounces of grain alcohol, and blended at high speed until the ginseng was practically dissolved. I poured this into a pint bottle, powdered roots and all, and set it in the cupboard for about a month, shaking it whenever I happened to think of it. I let it sit for a few days undisturbed, then carefully decanted the tincture off the settled roots. This liquid was a clear lemon-yellow in color, had a very slight odor of parsnips, and a drop of it on my tongue tasted first bitter, then sweet.

I tried adding a teaspoon of Ginseng Tincture to a wineglassful of Boneset Tea, with which I was experimenting at the time, and it didn't make that bitter brew taste any worse, and may have added to its medicinal benefits. A teaspoonful of this tincture added to a cup of coffee or tea makes a drinkable mixture and was probably doing all sorts of wonderful things for my health, of which I was totally unaware. This tincture could, no doubt, be added to the afternoon cocktail, in which I do not indulge, in place of commercial bitters.

Such a cocktail should about average out—the ginseng prolonging your life about as much as the alcohol in the cocktail will shorten it.

I wanted to see if I could give my last two ginseng roots that semi-transparency for which the Chinese are willing to pay such high prices. One reference hinted that this might be achieved by steaming, so I put the two roots on a wire rack over boiling water and steamed them for an hour, without getting the desired result. I remembered that calamus root became clear when boiled in sugar syrup, so I combined 1 cup of water and 1 cup of sugar, and sure enough, when I had boiled the roots for a few minutes in this syrup they began to display the translucency I was seeking. When they looked clear enough to suit me, I drained them and dried them on waxed paper for several days. I'm almost sure this is not the process used by Chinese druggists, but it made the little roots look good. I was afraid some of the expensive medical virtues had leached into the syrup, so I kept it and used it to sweeten sumach-ade and wild fruit juices.

A small bit of this Candied Ginseng was not at all bad to chew on. Besides being sweet, it had a bitter-aromatic flavor that one could learn to like if one could afford such expensive habits. Again, my chief pleasure in this root came from the knowledge that I was chewing on a substance for which a rich Chinese would pay ten times the price of gold.

While experimenting with ginseng, I talked a lot about the virtues the Chinese seemed to find in this drug, and I did not realize how much this talk had impressed my wife until the phone rang and she answered it. It was my agent calling from New York to give us the exceedingly cheering news that two of my books were doing far better than anyone had ever hoped, and assuring us that any financial worries we might have were about over. My wife, who had to teach school the first fourteen years of our married life so that I could afford the luxury of writing, was overjoyed. She excused herself for a minute, ran to the kitchen, then came back, picked up the phone and said, "I just went to the kitchen to get some of Euell's life-prolonging ginseng to chew on. If we are going to have that kind of money, I want to be around to enjoy it as long as I can."

26. How to Eat a Rose

R OSES are easily the best-known of all flowers. They grow around the world, from Greenland to Tasmania, from Lapland to Timbuktu, and from cold Siberia to southern India. There are dozens of species of wild rose, and more than 10,000 cultivated varieties. They have been portrayed by artists and celebrated by poets more than all other flowers put together. Everyone appreciates roses for their beauty and fragrance, but how many know that roses are also highly regarded for their flavor and food value in many parts of the world? Roses can be made into many delicious and luxurious dishes, ranging from condiments and flavorings through hearty main dishes and delightful beverages to delicate desserts and sublime jams and jellies. A rose is a rose is a rose— A rose by any other name— Gather ye rosebuds while ye may—but if you want roses in December, make some of the rose petals into a heavenly jam that can be stored away.

Uncooked Rose Petal Jam is astonishingly easy to make. I would like to think that it was sheer genius that caused me to get all the proportions right in my first attempt to make this fragrant ambrosia, but I know it was just blind luck. Gather freshly opened roses before the sun has distilled away too much of their ethereal flavor and fragrance. Wild roses are best, but any fragrant rose, provided it has not been sprayed with poisonous insecticides, will do. The deep-red roses give the color that I like best, but by using a different color for each batch you can soon make your jam cupboard resemble a well-planned rose garden.

The white base of the rose petal contains a bitter substance, and should be clipped away. This is not nearly the tedious job that it sounds. Grasp as many petals as you can hold between your finger and thumb, pull them from the rose and snip the white bases from all of them at once with a pair of shears. Prepare 1 cup of petals and put them into a blender with ¾ cup of water and the juice of 1 lemon. Blend until smooth, then gradually add 2½ cups sugar with the blender still running, and let it run until you are sure all the sugar has dissolved. Stir 1 package powdered pectin (Sure-Jell) into ¾ cup water, bring to a boil and boil hard for 1 minute, stirring constantly. Pour the pectin into the rose-sugar mixture and run the blender on slow until you are sure the pectin has been thoroughly incorporated with the other ingredients. Pour immediately into small sterilized jars with screw caps that will seal hermetically. Baby-food jars are ideal. I was amazed to find that fifteen minutes after I had gathered the roses, I was pouring the jam into the jars, and I hadn't hurried at all.

Allow the jars to stand at room temperature for about 6 hours, and the jam will be nicely jelled. It will keep for a month in the refrigerator, but if you want some for next winter, store it in the freezer. Then when the wind is howling about the eaves, and the sleet is pelting against the storm windows, you can bring a bright June day right into your kitchen by opening a jar of this rosy jam.

I have tried many other recipes for Rose Petal Jam, but this one is easily the best of them all. Being uncooked, all the color, flavor, and fragrance of the freshly blown rose is captured. Besides eating this jam in such obvious ways as spreading it on toast or hot biscuits, you can use it in preparing a number of exotic dishes that will enhance your reputation as a culinary artist. When I want to show off my prowess as a cook I sometimes make tiny muffins, flavoring the batter with a pinch of mace, a spice that enhances and complements the flavor of roses. When the muffins are nearly done, I slide the oven rack out part way, and keeping the muffins in partial heat, I make a small depression in the top of each one and fill it with rose jam. They are then returned to the oven to brown the muffins lightly and glaze the jam, then served hot, each muffin displaying a bright and tasty jewel in its crown.

Sometimes, too, I make thin French pancakes, quickly spread them with rose jam, and roll up each cake. Don't sprinkle these with powdered sugar, as so many cookbooks recommend; it looks too much as if the cook had spilled flour on them. Put a dollop of rose-colored whipped cream on each rolled-up pancake, or, even better, make a slight depression in the top of each rolled cake, put a teaspoon of

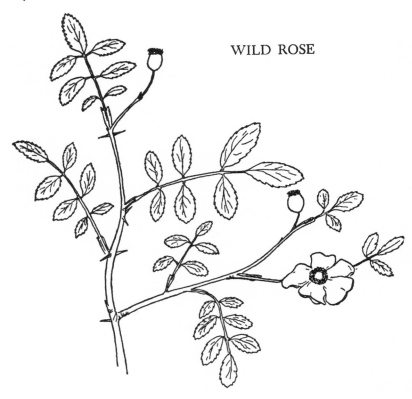

WILD ROSE

good cognac in each depression, set them afire, and bear the dish to the table in a blaze of glory.

Don't think that rose petals are good only for making jam. When I want to impress an overnight guest with an unusual breakfast, I make a Rose Omelet. Break 8 eggs into the blender, season with 1 level teaspoon celery salt and a pinch of marjoram, then add ½ cup of clean petals from freshly plucked roses. Blend at medium speed until the eggs are fluffy and the petals practically liquefied. Every good cook knows that a perfect omelet lies fully as much in the cooking as in the ingredients. Even a slightly scorched omelet isn't fit to eat. Pour the mixture into a greased pan over medium heat. If you have the heat just right, the bottom will be lightly browned when the top is just set. Make a crease across the top with a spatula, fold the omelet over and slide it onto a plate without trying to lift it, and it won't break apart. Decorate the omelet with a bright trail of paprika, and garnish the dish with dewy rosebuds. The rose petals in this omelet not only give it a spectacular color, but are actually good, and will be appreciated by anyone whose sense of taste is not overpowered by his prejudices. With a dish of Canadian bacon, this is a breakfast that can be set before the most discriminating gourmet with no apologies.

Candied Rose Petals are a delight to the eye and a joy to the tongue. Prepare the petals as for jam, plucking them from the rose in bunches and snipping off the white bases. Mix the white of 1 egg with 1 tablespoon water, dip each petal in this liquid and place the petals convex side up on a paper towel, to drain. When the excess liquid has drained off, but the petals are still evenly dampened, sprinkle both sides with granulated sugar. Shake off excess sugar and place the petals on waxed paper to dry for about 12 hours. Stored in a covered container in the refrigerator, Candied Rose Petals will keep their color and fragrance for about a month. Bring out a dish of these brightly colored petals instead of the usual after-dinner mints. They are not only beautiful, fragrant, and tasty, but, according to the ancient herbalist Culpepper, this confection is "a very good cordial against faintings, swoonings, weakness and trembling of the heart, strengthens a weak stomach, promotes digestion and is a very good preservative in the time of infection." What more could you ask of a few easily made Candied Rose Petals?

An even better candy is called Harem Kisses. Clip the white ends from red rose petals until you have 2 cups of prepared petals. Put these into your electric blender with just enough water, about a half-cup, so they will blend. Blend at high speed until they are reduced to a semiliquid mass. Add ½ pint of heavy cream, mix well, then gradually add powdered sugar until the whole is a doughlike mass that can be kneaded. Knead on a cutting board, adding more powdered sugar if necessary. Pat out flat, cover with a damp cloth, and allow it to stand for at least an hour. Shape into small pieces with the hands, topping each piece with a shelled pistachio nut.

Rose Water is a fragrant, flavorful liquid that is rich in ancient lore. Baptisms were formerly performed with rose water, and it is used in purification ceremonies to wash and perfume the temples and mosques of the East. The ancient Romans used Rose Water in their food, wine, and mixed drinks, and the very wealthy sometimes filled their fountains with this fragrant fluid. Rose Water has had an honored place in medicine since ancient days and is still used by the modern druggist for its healing properties and to impart a pleasant odor to pharmaceutical preparations. It is the favorite cosmetic of millions of Eastern women, and in the West it still enters into the composition of eyewashes, hand lotions, cold creams, and a well-known mouthwash.

All directions I can find for making Rose Water read about the same, and all call for distilling the volatile flavors and fragrances from fresh rose petals mixed with water. Such directions are all very well for a chemist with a laboratory in the back room, or a moonshiner with a still in the cellar, but they leave you and me wondering what to do. By experimenting I have improvised a perfectly workable still using nothing but ordinary kitchen utensils available to the average housewife. You will need a fairly deep pot, with a dome-shaped lid, a few ordinary cereal bowls, and some kind of rack that will hold a bowl away from the bottom of the pot as you cook. UNDER NO CIRCUMSTANCES used galvanized ware, or you will distill a poisonous product.

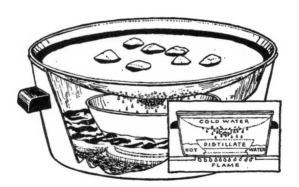

A DRIP STILL

I made my bowl rack out of an ordinary tuna-fish can. I cut off both ends, and punched a few holes in the sides so steam wouldn't get trapped inside and upset my bowl. I set this rack exactly in the center of the pot, poured in 1 quart of boiling water, then added 1 pound of rose petals and set the bowl on top of the improvised rack with 1 ice cube in the bowl. Then I inverted the dome-shaped lid, dumped a tray of ice cubes in it, filled it almost to the brim with cold water, set the pot on medium-high heat, and my still was in operation. The steam, containing the volatile flavors and aromas of the roses, strikes the cold lid, condenses, runs to the center of the lid, and drops into the bowl. The ice cube in the bowl is to prevent the more ethereal flavors, which evaporate below the boiling point of water, from revolatilizing.

This is really a very efficient little still, and the bowl will probably fill faster than you expect. Be sure to remove the bowl before the ice cube has completely melted, slipping in a cool bowl containing a new ice cube. Take no more than one cup of Rose Water from each batch, for after that you would be getting pretty weak stuff with very little flavor or aroma. If you want more Rose Water, gather more flowers and run off several batches. If all this work scares you, you can buy Rose Water from a druggist.

When you have a supply of this magic elixir, what should you do with it? In India, Rose Water is used to flavor soft drinks, sherbets, ice cream, cakes, and many other delicacies. In Turkey, a bottle of Rose Water appears on the table in lieu of catsup or savory sauce. The Arabs call Rose Water "dew of Paradise," and use it in glazing roasting fowls. This really transforms an ordinary chicken into a bird-of-paradise, and is worth a trial. To make the Glaze, mix together 3 tablespoons honey, 2 tablespoons melted butter, and 1 tablespoon Rose Water. Paint the whole outside of the bird with this mixture just before you put it in the oven, using a pastry brush. Any that is left can be painted on as you baste the roasting fowl.

To make a Seafood Sauce that does something for oysters, fish, scallops, and many other seafood dishes, mix 1 part lemon juice, 1 part melted butter, and 1 part Rose Water. Used discreetly, Rose Water can work magic in rice puddings, custards, and gelatin desserts. In Persia, there is a belief that if a woman gives an erring lover or husband some food containing Rose Water, he will thereafter be faithful to her. If American women ever accept this belief, it will send the consumption of Rose Water soaring.

To make Rose Wafers, blend ½ cup butter and ½ cup sugar. Add 1 well-beaten egg, ¾ cup flour, and a pinch of salt. Mix well, add 1 tablespoon Rose Water, work until smooth, then drop by teaspoonfuls on a well-greased cookie sheet and bake at 375° for about 10 minutes. These are really good!

I found several recipes for Rose Syrup made of dried rose petals, but found I cared little for this product. I later made some Rose-Water-flavored syrup that I liked very much. Mix together 2 cups sugar, 1 cup light corn syrup and ¾ cup water, and simmer for 20 minutes. When cool, add ¼ cup Rose Water, 1 teaspoon lemon juice, and enough red food coloring to give it a rosy tint. Pour into sterilized bottles with tight-fitting caps and store in a dark place.

This syrup not only goes well with pancakes and waffles, but also makes a delicious sauce for puddings, or topping for ice cream. To make a Rosy Soda put 2 tablespoons Rose Syrup in the bottom of a tumbler, add a scoop of vanilla ice cream, fill the glass with plain soda, and stir. When making Broiled Grapefruit, put a tablespoon of Rose Syrup in the center of each half just before you place them under the broiler. A clever cook will find many other uses for Rose Syrup and Rose Water.

Rose hips are better known as food than is the flower. I imagine most American housewives have at least heard of rose hips and their almost unbelievable vitamin C content, but I know very few cooks who actually use them. The hip is the fruit of the rose, a rather peculiar fruit, botanically, for it is formed by a swelling of the end of the stem which reaches up and encloses the seeds. They vary in size from species to species, from the tiny bird-shot size of the *Rosa multiflora* to the huge plum-sized hips of the *Rosa rugosa*. They are usually green during summer, turning orange, and finally bright-red, in the fall. For the very best hips, they should be gathered shortly after they turn bright-red, for later they develop a bothersome silkiness about the seeds. The larger varieties are more tasty, less tedious, and generally higher in vitamin content.

There is hardly any other food that is comparable with rose hips in vitamin C content. We think of oranges as rich in this vitamin, but a single cup of pared rose hips may contain as much vitamin C as 10 to 12 *dozen* oranges. In England, during the last war, there was a great shortage of citrus fruits, and the civilian population, the women, and the Boy Scouts turned out and picked thousands of tons of rose hips. At about the same time it was discovered that B vitamins could be processed from spent brewery hops, and some wag remarked that nutritionally England was getting by on its hips and hops. These rose hips were not, however, made into palatable delicacies by English housewives, but were pressed into pills to be sold in drugstores.

Very few American cooks seem to know how to prepare rose hips so they are really palatable. One cookbook, written by a vitamin-conscious nutritionist, recommends that the hips be cooked, then soaked in the cooking water, and that one takes three tablespoons of the cooking water per day. Ugh! The rose hip is a fruit, and not a bad fruit, either, so why make a disagreeable medicine of it?

In Northern Europe, from Germany to Lapland, rose hips were eaten purely for enjoyment, long before the word "vitamin" was coined. I turned to these Europeans in my search for good rose hip recipes. A German student promised to send me a recipe for rose hip jam when she returned to Germany, and she did, but it directed that the fruit and sugar be mixed together and *stirred for three hours*. I am inordinately interested in unusual foods, but I'm not *that* much interested. However, I wondered if I could make my trusty blender take over part of that muscular effort, and finally developed the following simple recipe.

To make Rose Hip Jam, prepare the hips by cutting off both the stem and the blossom ends, making a slit down the side of each hip and removing the seeds. Put 1 cup of prepared hips, ¾ cup water, and the juice of 1 lemon in the blender and blend until perfectly smooth. Gradually add 3 cups sugar, running the blender all the time. Blend together for about 5 minutes more, so all the sugar is completely dissolved. Stir 1 package powdered pectin in ¾ cup water, bring to a boil, and boil hard for 1 minute. Pour this into the blender and blend for 1 minute more. Pour immediately into small, sterilized screw-cap jars and store in the refrigerator. If it is to be kept for more than a month, store it in the freezer. Being uncooked, all the rich vitamin C content is retained, and a tablespoon of this really tasty jam will give you your minimum daily requirement of vitamin C. Isn't that better than swallowing a pill or taking medicine from a tablespoon?

A recipe for Rose Hip Soup was given to me by a Swedish school teacher to whom I shall remain eternally grateful. American housewives should get better acquainted with these Scandinavian fruit soups, which can be served hot or cold, as an appetizer at the beginning of a meal, or as a dessert at its close. They are very economical, wholesome, and easy to make, and a bowl of bright fruit soup can turn a very ordinary meal into a feast. They can be made of berries, cherries, and many other fruits, but for the very maximum in health benefits, make fruit soup of rose hips.

You don't need to seed the hips to be used for fruit soup. Use 2 cups of fresh rose hips and a quart of water, and boil until the hips are tender, then put through a sieve to remove the seeds and skins. Add enough water to make one quart again, stir in ½ cup sugar, and return it to the heat. Mix 1 tablespoon cornstarch into a smooth paste with a little water and stir this in. Cook a few minutes until it thickens slightly and looks clear. This is already a very good soup, served as is, but if you want to be really festive, stir in a jigger of Cherry Heering just before dishing it up, and float a spoonful of sour cream on each serving. It is excellent, and remember, with each spoonful you are being fortified with vitamin C to protect you against infections and deficiency diseases. A clever housewife will discover ways to add rose hips to ordinary jams, fruit sauces, and other dishes, not only giving her family good food but giving them buoyant health as well.

No wonder an ancient herbalist once wrote that the use of roses in cookery "Maketh a man merrie and joyful, putteth away all melancholie and madness." Try some of these rose recipes on a grouchy spouse.

27. Hawthorn or Red Haw

(*Crataegus*, many species)

THE HAWTHORN is a close relative of the apple, and that is about all one can say of this genus with certainty. Although it is not at all hard to recognize, once a few species have been closely observed, it is the most confusing tree in existence to try to describe, and it is the absolute despair of the taxonomist who tries to arrange the almost unlimited number of species into some logical classification. Hawthorns grow throughout Europe, North Africa, the nontropical parts of Asia, and in North America from well up in Canada, down to Mexico. There are from two hundred to nine hundred species, depending upon who is doing the counting. The best story I ever heard on the taxonomical confusion that surrounds this genus was told to me by Dr. Alfred Schuyler, the Chairman of Botany at the Academy of Natural Sciences in Philadelphia. He said a staff taxonomist was examining two specimens of *Crataegus* and found such wide and significant differences between them that he unhesitatingly placed them in two different species, then, on examining the collector's notes, made the embarrassing discovery that they were two specimens from opposite sides of the same tree.

There is hardly a thing one can say about hawthorn without immediately qualifying the statement. Some are shrubs no more than three feet high at maturity, but others are good-sized trees up to thirty feet in height with a trunk up to a foot in diameter near the base. Characteristic of this genus are the strong, fierce thorns from one to five inches in length, but some southern species are completely unarmed. The attractive clusters of five-petaled flowers are white, all but those few that are red or pink. The fruits are like tiny apples, except that on some species or varieties they are oval or pear-shaped. The fruit is a bright, glossy red, but occasionally one finds a tree with orange or yellow fruit, and one Far Western species has fruit that is black. On some trees the fruit is smaller than peas, and on others the haws may be an inch long. There may be one hard stone in some varieties and four to five in others. The fruit from one tree may have almost no flesh, and, from another, have a thick pulp between the stones and the tough outer skin. As to the quality of the fruit, it has been described as "too astringent to be considered edible," but an English botanist, William Wood, writing on the wild fruits of New England, only a few years after the landing of the Pilgrim Fathers, said, "the white thorne affords hawes as bigge as an English Cherrie, which is esteemed above a Cherrie for his goodnesse and pleasant-nesse to the taste." I have found a great many red haws that fit the former description and a very few that approached the latter one.

If you are interested only in herbal home remedies, probably the first hawthorn you encounter will serve, for the more astringent the berries the more potent they are medicinally. A decoction of the ripe fruit is used to cure sore throats and as a gentle corrective for diarrhea. Crush 1 cup of the berries, boil with 1 cup of water for 10 minutes, then strain and sweeten the juice to taste with honey. Take a table-spoonful at a time for sore throat, or a wineglassful at a time for diarrhea. The bark of the hawthorn has been said to be a cardiac tonic, useful in organic and functional heart troubles, but as I could find no recipe or dosage for this, and as I did not feel my heart needed a tonic, I did not experiment with the bark.

If you are more interested in this fruit as food than as medicine, and wish to taste red haws at their very best, I can only advise that you taste the fruit from every hawthorn you see until you find a tree that bears good fruit. When I was a boy I knew where all the best haws grew in my neighborhood, and I don't remember going to any great trouble to acquire that knowledge, but now they seem very hard to find. Last fall I determined to find the best red haws that grow in central Pennsylvania, where I now live. There are hawthorns of many species and varieties growing everywhere in this area, but on most of them the fruit is very poor in quality. Helping me with this project was an 11-year-old girl who is one of the keenest students of nature that I know. We set out one Saturday morning in late September when the haws were red and glossy and spent the entire day

HAWTHORN

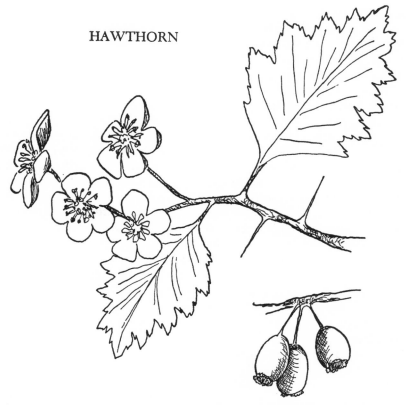

driving from place to place where I had noticed hawthorn trees growing, sampling the fruit from as many different trees as possible. Most of the haws we tried were not worth picking, some promised very good jams and jellies, and a few were perfectly edible raw, but none of them would have been described as delicious by anyone with normal taste and reasonable honesty. At the end of the day, my small companion cleverly summed up her opinion of red haws by paraphrasing a nursery rhyme, "When they are good, they are not very good, and when they are bad, they are horrid."

However, we picked several pailfuls of the best fruit we found, and that evening we discovered the true worth of the red haw. It makes excellent jelly and marmalade. We made several batches of both Haw Jelly and Haw Marmalade that fall, and thoroughly enjoyed eating it the following winter. We even gave away a few jars as Christmas presents to very special friends. Incidentally, the jelly has exactly the same medicinal value as the decoction described above, and a very pleasant way of treating a sore throat is simply to eat some of this delicious jelly.

To make Haw Jelly, crush 3 pounds of the fruit, add 4 cups of water, bring it to a boil, cover the kettle and let it simmer for 10 minutes, then strain the juice through a jelly bag and discard the spent pulp, seeds, and skins. If red haws are not too ripe, they will furnish ample pectin for jelly making, but if they are very ripe, add 1 package powdered pectin to the strained juice. We felt our juice could stand more acid, so we added the juice of 2 lemons. We put just 4 cups of this juice in a very large saucepan and brought it to a boil, then added 7 cups of sugar and very soon after it came to a boil again, it showed a perfect jelly test. (This test is performed by dipping up a very little of the juice in a cooking spoon, waving it around until it has slightly cooled, then pouring it from the edge of the spoon. If it is going to jell when cool, it will betray that fact at this time by the last few drops running together and sheeting off the spoon in a semi-jelled glob.) We poured our jelly into sterilized straight-sided, half-pint jars and sealed them with sterilized two-piece metal dome lids to avoid having to use paraffin.

To make Haw Marmalade, we cooked some haws in very little water for about 15 minutes, then forced them through a conical colander, or ricer, with a wooden pestle. For each batch we used 1½ cups of the strained haw pulp and the juice and peels from 1 lemon and 1 orange. The juice was stirred directly into the pulp, but the peels required some processing. First we shaved away about half of the white material on the inner sides of the peels, snipped them into fine shreds with a pair of kitchen shears. Next we put them in a saucepan with 2 cups of water and about ⅛ teaspoon of soda, and boiled them for 20 minutes, then drained and added these cooked peels to the other ingredients. One package of powdered pectin was stirred into the mixture, it was returned to the fire, and as soon as it boiled we added 5 cups of sugar. When it regained a boil, we let it boil hard for 1 minute, then poured it into the sterilized jars and sealed them. To one batch of marmalade, I added ½ teaspoon of powdered rosemary. I like the marmalade best of all my recipes for this fruit.

28. The Useful Chickweed
(*Stellaria media*)

ALTHOUGH the chickweed is detested by farmers and gardeners, I love this little plant and can hardly bring myself to hoe it out of my vegetable garden. This is one plant that is readily available to nearly every reader of this book, for it is found around the world, from Greenland to Tierra del Fuego, from Lapland to Capetown, and from Siberia to Tasmania. Wherever Europeans have gone this plant has followed, becoming a common weed in all countries. Chickweed can be found and used any time it is not covered with snow, and from New York southward it can be found in bloom every month of the year.

Chickweed is so common that we tend to overlook it, except on well-tended lawns, but this little plant is well worth a close examination by anyone at all interested in herbs. The tender, juicy, pale-green stems are much branched and slightly swollen at the joints and may reach a length of more than a foot, but are so thin and weak that they are usually procumbent; chickweed seldom rises more than a few inches off the ground unless it is growing so thickly that the plants support one another. The leaves are in opposite pairs placed every inch or so along the stem. Each leaf is about a half-inch long and a quarter-inch across, tender and succulent, egg-shaped with a sudden little point on the outer end. The new-born leaves appear sessile, or stalkless, but the lower end of each young leaf gradually elongates into a flat leafstalk about as long as the leaf itself. For certain identification, examine the plant under low-power magnification, such as a reading glass. You will see a single line of tiny hairs running up one side of the stem. When this line reaches a pair of leaves it continues up the opposite side of the stem to the next pair, alternating the side of the stem on which it chooses to travel at each pair of leaves.

The flowers are only about a quarter-inch across, and occur singly in the axils of the upper leaves. They are white, star-shaped with five petals, each petal deeply cleft at its outer end. These flowers open about midmorning on sunny days, but on cloudy or rainy days they may not open at all. The chickweed is a good illustration of "sleep" in plants, for not only do the flowers close at night, but the paired leaves approach one another so their upper surfaces fold over the tender, developing buds in their axils, and the outermost pair of fully developed leaves envelop the terminal bud as though trying to protect the tender, growing shoot.

Chickweed receives its common name because young chickens and small birds love it, eagerly eating both the leaves and the seeds, and they thrive on it. It is also eminently edible by human beings, and it could restore health to millions of malnourished people throughout the world if they would only use it. I know a family of health-food enthusiasts in southern Pennsylvania who eat chickweed nearly every day that it is available, and that means most of the year. They liquefy chickweed, along with a number of other assorted herbs, wild and domestic, to make what they call Green Drink, which is their favorite beverage. Chickweed is also chopped into the tossed salads they love so well and is mixed with other greens to make the cooked vegetable dishes to which they are addicted. Even the broth from these cooked greens is not wasted; it goes into the green drink. There are seven people in this family, from preschool to middle-aged; they take no medicine, all enjoy buoyant health, sickness being almost unknown among them, and none of them is overweight. They could easily afford any kind of food they happen to want, but they refuse to abandon their green-herb diet, not only because it gives them such superb health and bounding energy, but because they have actually come to prefer these tastes.

Chickweed has long been used as a cooked vegetable. I find a whole series of herbals stating that boiled chickweed is as good as spring spinach. They probably picked up the idea from some now-forgotten source rather than learning from actual experience, which I consider inexcusable laziness, for anyone can find enough chickweed for a trial. It really tastes very little like spinach, so I don't consider the comparison a valid one. I eat both spinach and chickweed, like them both, and never think of one as a substitute for the other. Boiled chickweed is mild and bland with a slight herbal flavor. I like it better when it is mixed with stronger-flavored greens, like watercress, wild mustard, shepherds-purse, peppergrass, or winter-cress. Those who prefer mild and almost tasteless greens may enjoy plain boiled chickweed, but to me its flat taste seems to cry out for a little of the pungent pepperiness of the *Cruciferae*.

Chickweed is so tender that it cooks almost instantly, and it should always be short-cooked to preserve the maximum amount of its health-giving nutrients. To make Chickweed and Greens, I always use about 2 parts chickweed and 1 part stronger greens. The stronger greens are put on first, covered with boiling water, and cooked about 10 minutes; then the chickweed is added, and after the water has regained a boil it is cooked about 2 minutes more. Drain, but do not throw away that cooking-water. Chop the greens right in the cooking pot, using kitchen shears; season with salt, butter, a little pepper sauce, and some finely chopped raw onion. Sprinkle each serving with some crumbled crisp bacon. This makes a hearty and palatable vegetable dish that requires no apologies.

It is hard to give a recipe for the Green Drink that my friends make, for it is seldom constructed twice the same way. The mother of this family may put as many as 15 different kinds of green herbs in the blender at once, guided by her extensive knowledge of nutrition and an amazing taste-memory. A sample Green Drink might be made by using chiefly chickweed and dwarf mallow leaves, but then she would probably add sheep-sorrel, a little watercress, some mint, chives or green onion, winter-cress, thyme, rue, parsley, comfrey (her kitchen windowsill is lined with herbs growing in flowerpots, which she adds to her wild herbs), and almost any green garden vegetables that happen to be in season. To this blend she will add any broth or vegetable cooking-water she has on hand, a little lemon juice or cider vinegar, and a touch of honey. She uses no salt, claiming that there is enough sodium chloride found naturally in the herbs and vegetables she uses to furnish all of this mineral the body needs, but I like a little added salt.

In my own experiments with Green Drink I have sometimes cheated by adding things that were not green, such as diced apples or carrots, a fresh radish or two, dill, anise, or caraway seeds, shelled hickory nuts or black walnuts, orange juice, cider, and even sometimes peeled halves of tree-ripened peaches or apricots. All these extra flavorings worked, some better and some worse, but none made the conglomeration undrinkable.

I think the palatability of a well-made Green Drink lies in the combination of opposite flavors. To compare it with a far less healthful drink, it is like the Irish tourist's description of the American cocktail. He said, "They put in whiskey to make it strong and water to make it weak, lemon to make it sour and sugar to make it sweet, spice to make it hot and ice to make it cold, shake it all up together, say, 'Here's to you,' then drink it themselves." To make a good Green Drink put in some strong flavors and some weak ones, something sour and something sweet, a pungent herb and a cooling one, some bitter flavors and some bland ones, something spicy and something mild. Simply fill your blender jar with these selected herbs, cover them with water, broth, vegetable stock, fruit juice, tomato juice, or a mixture of any or all of them, add lemon or vinegar and a little honey, blend at high speed until the herbs are practically liquefied, then pour into tumblers and serve immediately. Green Drink should never be made ahead as storage robs it of nutrients and debases the flavor, so drink it while it is fresh and frothy.

Besides using chickweed as a green vegetable and adding it to Green Drink, you can eat it raw. A salad of pure chickweed is not inedible if properly dressed, but it is much improved by including some better-flavored herbs, wild or domestic, and a little onion. Again, no recipe can be given; just add some chickweed to almost any tossed salad you are making, and I think you will be pleased with the result. I know your health will benefit.

I found chickweed listed as a medicinal herb in every herbal I consulted. It has a reputation as a demulcent, emollient, refrigerant, antiscorbutic, and as a low-calorie vegetable for a reducing diet. The old medical term *antiscorbutic* can now be translated, "a source of vitamin C." To get the full vitamin benefits from chickweed, no medicine is necessary. Just eat chickweed salads and drink Green Drink, and you will never be in danger of contracting scurvy, which is a vitamin C deficiency disease. Most green vegetables and fresh fruits contain vitamin C, but chickweed was formerly a very important antiscorbutic because it could be obtained during the winter when scurvy was most prevalent and when most other green vegetables were unobtainable.

Eating boiled chickweed and drinking the broth has long been an old wives' remedy for obesity. If this common plant will actually help dieters to shed pounds, it will attract more attention among moderns for this use than for any other. I'm sure it will work if the chickweed greens and juice are not merely taken in addition to your regular meals, but substituted for some of the calorie-laden starches, sweets, and fats you usually eat. It may be no better and no worse for this purpose than some other low-calorie, high-vitamin foods, but it is far cheaper. If you don't already know where chickweed can be had for the taking, a walk through the countryside in search of it will cause you to lose even more pounds.

Probably the greatest use the old herbalists found for chickweed was as an external poultice used in treating boils, inflammation, indolent ulcers, carbuncles, and external abscesses. The fresh herb was covered with boiling water, then allowed to cool enough to be applied to the affected part; it was bound loosely to the sore and changed often. They also recommended that the affected part be washed frequently in the water in which the herb had steeped. These uses lead one to suspect that chickweed may have some antibiotic activity that science has not yet discovered. If an antibiotic agent is there, it may soon be discovered by the scientists who are exploring these old herbal remedies in search of new antibiotics. As one old astrological herbalist says of chickweed, "it is a fine, soft, pleasing herb, under the dominion of the Moon," and another says, "in a word it comforteth, digesteth, defendeth and suppurateth very notably."

29. The Versatile Viburnums:

BLACK-HAW, STAGBUSH, OR FALSE CRAMP BARK

(Viburnum prunifolium)

THE BLACK-HAW is a shrub or small tree that offers the nature-lover outstanding beauty, interesting home remedies, and one of the sweetest of all wild fruits. In the spring, just as the leaves are unfolding, the black-haw produces gorgeous clusters of white flowers, two to four inches across, resembling those of the well-known domestic snowball. The individual blossoms that compose this cluster have flat corollas, deeply five-lobed, and five stamens. Nature offers few sights more beautiful than a haw bush in full bloom. This shrub received its specific name, *prunifolium*, because its leaves closely resemble those of the plum tree. These leaves grow in opposite pairs, are sharply and finely toothed at the margins, and are from one to two inches long and about half as wide, oval in shape, and rather bluntly pointed. The flowers are followed by clusters of green berries that become bright-red by late summer and gradually turn blue-black, or purple-black, with a dusty bloom, by late autumn. The individual berries are about a half-inch long, oval in outline, and slightly flattened, with a dark, very sweet pulp and an oval, flat stone.

It is hard to comment on the quality of this fruit, for it varies tremendously from one district to another, and even from one bush to another. All are very sweet, some are fat and pulpy, but others have a pulp so thin as to be almost nonexistent. The flavor ranges from bland to delicious. Those who deprecate the quality of this really excellent wild fruit simply have not yet tasted black-haws at their best. Bushes bearing good fruit are found from New England to Florida and west to Texas. It was in Texas that I first made the acquaintance of this natural sweetmeat. I was nine years old and was visiting some cousins in the Red River Valley. They knew where the finest haws grew and passed up bushes with mediocre or poor fruit without a second glance. I thought the haws from their favorite bushes the finest wild fruit I had ever tasted, and I still like them, not for cooking, or dessert at the table, but to eat directly from the bush, in brisk, frosty fall weather. Like Thoreau's wild apples, I think the black-haw should come labeled, "To be eaten in the wind."

It seems strange to me that more effort has not been made to domesticate the black-haw, for it shows great promise. There is great seedling variation in the size, quantity, and quality of the fruit, and the best haws are excellent, though a bit seedy. Cultivation and selection would no doubt improve this fruit, and a skillful plant breeder might be able to induce the black-haw to hybridize with some of the closely related fruit-bearing viburnums, thus giving rise to still more varieties, any one of which might prove superior. If a valuable variety is ever developed, it will be easily propagated by rooted cuttings, air layering, or grafting.

I have tried cooking black-haws, but I can't point to any outstanding successes with this fruit. When boiled with some sugar and lemon peel, then put through a colander to remove the bothersome seeds, black-haws make a fair Fruit Sauce, but I can make a better one with ordinary prunes. Once, while camping with a deer-hunting party, I gathered some black-haws, squeezed the seeds from them, and added the sweet pulp to the cooked cereal we had for breakfast the next morning. It was quite good, with a flavor reminiscent of dates. However, what tastes wonderful when eaten around a campfire on a frosty dawn may show up rather poorly in the dining room, and, later, when I tried the same mixture for Sunday breakfast, it seemed banal and uninteresting. Until some Burbank tames and civilizes this wild sweet fruit I will enjoy it only on my outdoor jaunts and hikes, for it seems to resent being brought indoors before being eaten.

It is the dried bark of the stems of the black-haw that is used for herbal remedies. The easiest time to collect this bark is in the spring, about the time the shrub flowers, for then the sap is rising and the bark slips easily from the stems. Dry the bark indoors, then store it in a tight container; collect a new supply each year, for it loses strength with age. Formerly, the gathering and selling of this bark was a minor industry in some parts of our country, for it was widely used as an antispasmodic and could then be purchased in any drugstore. Because the bark of the closely related highbush-cranberry had already preempted the name "cramp bark," the bark of the blackhaw, which was similarly used, was called "false cramp bark." However, when it was discovered that the active principle in both these cramp barks was a bitter glucoside called *viburnin*, the barks were assayed for this drug, and it was found that the "false" cramp bark was three times as potent as the "true."

To make the home remedy, shave fine 1 ounce of the dried bark, cover with 1 pint of boiling water, and steep until the infusion has cooled. Strain, and take 1 tablespoonful of the liquid 3 times a day, before meals. This infusion was thought to prevent cramps of all kinds and was believed to be especially efficacious in preventing or allaying the pains that sometimes accompany menstruation. It was also used by pregnant women with a history of miscarriages, and was thought to enable such women to carry their babies to normal birth. For this purpose a pregnant woman would start taking the infusion about 5 weeks before trouble was expected and continue the recommended dosage of 1 tablespoonful, 3 times a day, until the danger period was passed. Modern medicine has been unable to discover any specific medical or physiological action by this infusion that could account for the results observed, and its use by professional practitioners has almost ceased, but many women still feel sure that this remedy enabled them to bear healthy, live babies after a heartbreaking series of miscarriages.

WILD-RAISIN
(V. *Lentago*)

Closely related to the black-haw is the wild-raisin, nannyberry, or sheepberry, which grows from Hudson Bay to New Jersey and west to Kansas. It, too, is a large shrub or small tree, sometimes reaching a height of thirty feet, but any specimen over fifteen feet tall is exceptional. Its leaves are larger than those of the black-haw, being two to four inches long and about half that in width. These leaves are

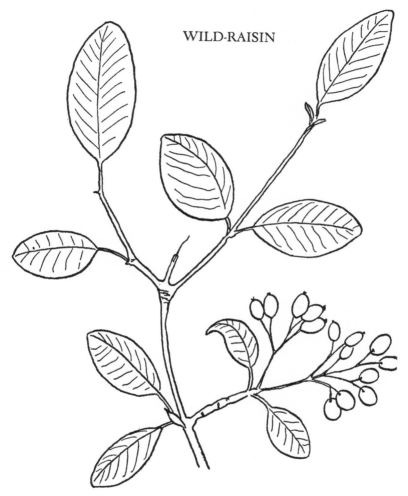

WILD-RAISIN

borne on leafstalks about an inch long, and these leafstalks have thin
membranous processes along each margin, and this wing margin is
one of the recognition features that help to distinguish the species.
The leaves are rounded at the base and rather abruptly pointed at the
apex, and the margins are finely and sharply toothed. The flower
clusters are two to four inches across and very attractive. They are
followed by clusters of ovoid, or egg-shaped, berries, each fruit about

half an inch long, green in summer, and turning directly to black on ripening, with no intermediate red stage as in the black-haw.

This fruit is also edible, and, like the black-haw, varies in size and quality from bush to bush. Some people prefer the wild-raisin to the black-haw, but to my taste they are never as good as the black-haw at its finest, although this may be because I did not know the berry as a child and therefore did not develop a taste for it. Commercial herb gatherers often mix the bark of this species with that of V. *prunifolium*, and since the drug buyers and users never seem to detect the substitution, we can assume that it has the same medicinal content as the bark of the black-haw.

WITHEROD
(V. *cassinoides*)

The witherod, or Appalachian tea, is another closely related species that grows in swamps and along streams from Newfoundland to Manitoba and south to New Jersey and Minnesota, and on south in the mountains to Georgia. It is a shrub, five to twelve feet high; the young shoots are covered with rusty scales, the opposite leaves, 1 to 3 inches long, are thick and obscurely veined; the margins are crenulate, or wavy, and either very finely toothed or smooth. The fruit is black with a bluish bloom, and much smaller than that of the two species described above. This fruit is more a nibble than a solid food, for the berries are about the size of small raisins and the stone is large. The thin pulp is very sweet and quite good-flavored, what there is of it, and since the little black berries often hang on the bush until far into the winter, I like to gather a pocketful as I hike across frozen swamps that are inaccessible in the summertime and nibble on them as I walk, spitting the seeds everywhere and no doubt starting new clumps of this interesting bush.

The leaves of this shrub have been used for tea, and it is sometimes called False Paraguay Tea. If the leaves are merely dried and used, the tea is a pretty poor beverage. I have found that if they are steamed over boiling water for a few minutes, then rolled between the fingers, allowed to stand in an open bowl overnight, then dried in an oven, the tea has a bright-amber color and a nice taste and is almost worth the work you have put into it. I don't know whether or not this tea will prevent cramps, as an infusion of the bark is supposed to do, but it seems a good, wholesome hot beverage and is worth drinking for its flavor alone.

THE HIGHBUSH-CRANBERRY, CRAMP BARK, OR GUELDER-ROSE
(V. *Opulus*)

The highbush-cranberry is a valuable wild plant yielding food, drink, medicine, and beauty, but it is not related to the cranberry. Neither is the almost identical guelder-rose of England a rose. They are tall shrubs reaching from six to ten feet in height, and they are related to the honeysuckle, the elderberry, and the black-haw. The Old World and New World kinds appear identical to the untrained eye, and one description will do for both. They are slender shrubs or small trees, a number sprouting from a single root, and they tend to form thickets along streams and in low, wet places. The bark is a pale ashy-brown, the leaves are opposite, toothed, and terminate in three pointed lobes of almost equal size. These leaves are two to three inches across and slightly resemble maple leaves. The attractive white flowers the bushes bear appear in showy clusters three to four inches across, with large sterile blossoms about the edge of the cluster and much smaller fertile ones near its center. These are followed later by bountiful clusters of bright-red berries, each fruit about one-third inch in diameter, that ripen in late summer, but soften and become better after being touched by frost, and will hang on the bushes all winter. Birds will eat these berries, but usually don't touch them until nearly spring, when other food becomes scarce.

V. *Opulus* has been hailed as a valuable medicinal plant since ancient days. Chaucer calls the fruit "gaitre berries" and lists them among the plants that "shal be for your hele" and recommends that you "picke hem right as they grow and eat hem in," an excellent way of being sure that you are taking full advantage of this berry's not inconsiderable vitamin C content.

Because it was only in this century that ascorbic acid was studied, isolated, analyzed, and named "vitamin C," we are apt to claim that this essential nutrient was discovered by modern research, but that is not so. Vitamin C was discovered the first time someone noticed that scurvy patients quickly recovered when fed certain fruits and vegetables, and this probably happened thousands of years ago. The ancients did not know vitamin C by name, but they did discover an imposing list of plants that were antiscorbutic, and I'm not at all sure that they were not ahead of us in prescribing freshly picked, wholesome food, rich in vitamin C, as a remedy for scurvy, rather than pills from the druggist.

Before the advent of vitamin pills, imported citrus fruits, bottled fruit juices, and frozen fresh vegetables, most vitamin C deficiencies occurred in winter, and this made V. *Opulus* an especially valuable plant, as its berries with their rich vitamin C content hang onto the bushes and stay fresh and edible all winter. Unfortunately, the Old World berries were too bitter to be really palatable, but many northern peoples ate them anyway, probably more for their health-giving benefits than for their flavor. In northern Europe and Asia, from England to Japan, these bitter berries have probably cured a million cases of scurvy, and prevented millions more.

When the first settlers came from the Old World to what is now northern United States and southern Canada, they found a shrub almost identical in appearance to the familiar guelder-rose, but with the characteristic bitter taste reduced to quite palatable levels. The pioneer housewives soon discovered that these berries would make excellent fruit juice, jelly, and sauces, which so closely resembled those made of cranberries, in both flavor and color, that the bush came to be known as the highbush-cranberry, although botanically it is entirely unrelated to the real cranberry.

Some botanists consider the American highbush-cranberry a separate species and call it V. *trilobum*, while others insist that it is only a variety of the European species and label it V. *Opulus*, variety *americanum*. This plant, with its palatable, debittered berries, is found from Newfoundland to British Columbia and south to New Jersey and Oregon. To further compound the confusion, the Old World V. *Opulus* has been planted as an ornamental, and has sometimes escaped to the wild over much of this same range. The only way the amateur herbalist can distinguish between the two is by taste; if the berries are too bitter to make good juice and jelly, it is the European variety. Fortunately, neither species is poisonous, and both kinds seem equally efficacious medicinally.

One reason I like highbush-cranberries is that they are so easy to pick, and I write this after having picked a half-bushel in 20 minutes, only yesterday. These shrubs often fruit so heavily that the upper limbs are weighed down, with each bright cluster of cherry-red berries seeming to beg to be broken off and dropped into a pail. Last night I made enough highbush-cranberry juice to give me a great many high C breakfast drinks this coming winter.

Highbush-Cranberry Juice is easily made. Fill a 6-quart kettle two-thirds full of berries and just cover with water. With a potato peeler, shave the outside colored part of an orange rind into the kettle, then add the juice of the orange. The orange peel and juice is to improve the aroma, and is quite necessary, as the guelder-rose doesn't smell like a rose. Both the flowers and the crushed berries of V. *Opulus* are ill-smelling to most noses, but the orange oil in the peel masks this bad smell, or rather, blends with the odor of the berries and transforms it into a bearable fragrance. Simmer the berries for about 3 minutes, then crush with a potato masher, stir to loosen any pulp that has stuck to the bottom, simmer 2 minutes more, then strain through a jelly bag or two thicknesses of cheesecloth. Reheat the juice just to boiling, then pour into sterilized bottles and seal with crown caps.

I first tried crushing the berries raw, but found they squirted bright-red juice all over me and my kitchen. A few minutes' simmering softens the skins, and the water covering prevents the juice from flying out of the kettle. The extra water doesn't matter, for even juice made this way is still too concentrated to be entirely palatable without dilution. This juice contains so much acid and other flavors that it must be treated like lemon juice or like the concentrated juices that you buy at the supermarket. Mixed with 2 parts water to 1 part juice, and sweetened to taste with sugar syrup, it makes a dandy "Cranberry" cocktail that is loaded with vitamins to protect your health. Even diluted in this fashion, it is still nearly as rich in vitamin C as freshly squeezed, undiluted, orange juice. So, drink to your own health in bright-colored, fine-tasting Highbush-Cranberry Juice.

To make a beautifully clear Highbush-Cranberry Jelly, prepare the juice exactly as directed above, strain it into a mixing bowl, and set it in the refrigerator overnight to settle. Next day carefully dip off 4 cups of juice, stir in 1 package commercial powdered pectin, and bring to a boil. The instant it boils, stir in 5 cups sugar, bring back to a boil, and boil hard for 1 minute, then pour into straight-sided, half-pint jars and seal with two-piece metal lids. This jelly has a full-bodied flavor that makes it go very well with meats or fowl, but it can also be eaten with hot biscuits, muffins or rolls, or just spread on an ordinary piece of toast.

HIGHBUSH-CRANBERRY

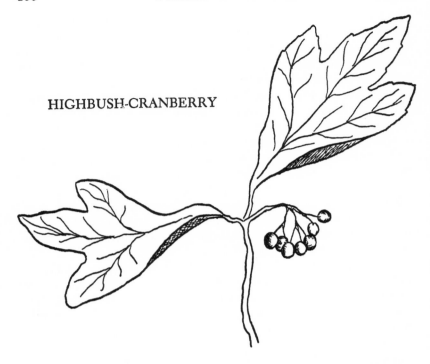

If you prefer a Fruity Highbush-Cranberry Sauce, cook the berries as directed for juice, not forgetting the orange and its peel, then, instead of straining it through a jelly bag, mash the fruit through a coarse colander to remove only the seeds. To four cups of the juicy pulp add 1 package commercial pectin, boil, add 5 cups sugar, and proceed exactly as in making the clear jelly.

While studying this plant, I kept running across reports that the Siberians used the berries from the Old World variety for making a fermented drink, but none of the references came up with a recipe. I was interested, because near my home, on the abandoned towpath of a long disused canal, European V. *Opulus* grows so thickly as to form a regular hedge, and it hurts me to see so many tons of the berries go to waste every year. True, these berries are very bitter, but I wondered if this bitterness might not be more palatable in wine than it is in food. We seem to enjoy a bitter flavor in alcoholic beverages, for we add bitters to a cocktail and hops to our beer. An attempt at making wine of these berries seemed worth a try. I made 2 gallons of juice as directed above, added 5 pounds of sugar, then, when it had cooled to lukewarm, I added a cake of yeast that was first dissolved in a cupful of the juice. This was poured into a crock and covered with a cloth. It fermented furiously for several days, then began to settle down, and in about 6 weeks it became quiet and clear. It was then siphoned off into half-gallon jugs that were stopped with wads of cotton.

After about 6 months I happened to think of this wine again and went to the cellar to inspect it. There was a brown sediment on the bottom of each jug, and above this sediment the wine was clear and bright. Already, it seemed drinkable to my taste, but I wanted to see what age would do for it, so I carefully siphoned it into green ginger ale bottles that I sealed with crown caps. The next year, at Christmas, I opened a bottle. It was exceedingly clear, of a beautiful color that one of my friends called a "tawny pink," and the taste—well, I like it, but I can't claim to be an expert on wines. The sugar apparently had not been totally converted to alcohol, for it was still slightly sweet. The bitter of the berries actually improved the flavor, rather than detracting from it. I thought it would be an excellent table wine to serve with meats, fowl, or fish, but my wife detested its flavor, and my friends seem about equally divided on its merits. Let's just say that it is a good wine if you happen to like it.

From what I have written, one would suppose that the fruit was the only useful part of V. *Opulus,* but most herbalists ignore the berries completely and write only about the wonderful medicinal properties of the bark. "Cramp bark," it is called, and once it appeared in the *U.S. Pharmacopoeia,* and it still is official in the *National Formulary.* It is listed as an antispasmodic, and its chief use has been as a uterine sedative to allay the pains that sometimes accompany the menstrual period. Its usefulness in this condition was apparently discovered independently by Europeans, Asiatic tribes, and American Indians. One of its common American names, dating from the days of early settler contact with the Indians, is "squawbush." However, this medicinal bark is not solely a woman's remedy, for it has been used as an antispasmodic in treating asthma, epilepsy, and convulsions, and even as a preventive of muscular cramps or "charley horses."

The best time to gather the bark is in the spring, when the rising sap causes it to peel easily. Left to itself, this shrub tends to grow too thickly, so cut out a few stems with an easy conscience, for your depredations will only cause the average clump to grow faster and fruit more profusely. Take the stems you cut to a shady place, sit down, and peel them in comfort. With a sharp pocketknife make a cut all around the stem, through the bark, every six inches, then slit each of these sections down one side and remove the bark by sliding your knife under it. Often these small sections of bark can be removed whole; they will curl back together as they dry, leaving you with quill-like tubes of bark. Dry the bark thoroughly in a warm room, then keep in a covered container until used. Renew your supply yearly, for it loses its strength with age.

The dried bark is nearly odorless, and the taste is astringent and decidedly bitter. Its active principle is a bitter glucoside called viburnin. I suspect that some of this same glucoside is contained in the fruit, for the bitter of the bark and the bitter of the berries, especially those of the European variety, are very similar in taste. Pharmacists manufacture tinctures and elixirs from this bark, but for home use it is usually taken as an infusion, or tea. A level tablespoon of the bark, cut fine, is covered with a pint of boiling water and allowed to infuse for half an hour, then strained. This is taken cold, a whiskey-glassful at a time, until the cramps disappear.

SQUASHBERRY
(V. *edule*)

For those who live farther north, there is a close relative of the highbush-cranberry that bears even better fruit. This is the squashberry, V. *edule*, which grows from Newfoundland to Alaska, coming south to northern New England, New York, and Pennsylvania, and has been reported from cool regions in Michigan, Wisconsin, and Minnesota. It is a straggling shrub, smaller than the highbush-cranberry, with smaller and less acid berries borne in somewhat smaller clusters. The leaves are opposite, as in all viburnums, and are even more maple-like than those of the highbush-cranberry. The berries are bright-red, and, when fully ripe, are very pleasant to the taste, even raw, for they are only mildly acid after being touched by the frost. They will never be popular as a fresh fruit because of the large flat stone, but they do make excellent juice, sauce, or jelly.

The juice is made exactly like that from highbush-cranberry, except that it needs no dilution before drinking. Just chill and sweeten to taste with sugar syrup. The jelly and sauce are made precisely like those of highbush-cranberry, but the flavor is milder and the products even better, if possible. As far as I know, this fruit has never been tested to determine its vitamin C content, but when it is, I'll wager that it will be found to be very rich in this protective vitamin.

30. Those Marvelous Mallows

(*Althea* and *Malva* species)

T HE MOST important mallow, from the herbalist's point of view,
is the marsh-mallow, *Althea officinalis*. It is not native to America,
and has a very limited range. The first marsh-mallow was probably
brought to this country in earth used as ship ballast, and the plant
has never ventured far from the sea, but it is well established and
abundant in many salt marshes and near tidal rivers along the Eastern
Seaboard. The root is perennial, and from it, each spring, come several sparingly branched stems that grow to three or four feet tall. The
short-stalked leaves are three-to-five-lobed, about two inches across
and three inches long, toothed at the margins, slightly resembling a
maple leaf in outline—though far different in texture, the mallow leaf
being covered on both sides with a fine, soft down. The flowers,
which bloom through August and September, are five-petaled, about
two inches across, pale pink in color, and by their form readily betray
their relationship to the hibiscus and hollyhock, even to the amateur
eye.

Although the plant is not widely known in this country, the term
marshmallow is familiar to everyone, for this herb long ago gave its
name to a puffy confection that was ancestral to the marshmallows
that children love to roast over campfires. Originally, marshmallows
were made of a mucilaginous extract of real marsh-mallow root, and
were considered more a medicine than a sweetmeat. They were chiefly
used as a very pleasant method of treating a cough, sore throat, or

bronchitis. Modern marshmallows are made of egg albumin, syrup, starch, gum, and flavoring, and contain no marsh-mallow whatever.

The perennial roots are thick, long, and tapering, with a yellowish-white corky layer on the outside, and the inside white and fibrous. The whole plant, and especially the root, abounds in a bland, sweetish mucilage that gives mallow its medicinal and nutritional virtues. The root also contains starch, pectin, oil, sugar, asparagine, calcium, glutinous matter, and cellulose.

These roots are edible and were mentioned in the Book of Job in the Old Testament, making this one of the first wild-food plants to be written about. In Chapter XXX, verse 4, Job is complaining that he has fallen so far from his formerly honorable estate that even the semi-wild ne'er-do-wells who live in the wilderness and "cut up mallows . . . for their meat" are now deriding him. One writer of the 16th century says that the poorer inhabitants of Egypt, Syria, Greece, and Armenia sometimes subsisted for weeks together on wild herbs, and that mallow was one of their favorites. These literary mentions of mallow as a famine food do not especially recommend it, except in emergencies, and I was elated to discover that those lusty gourmets, the Romans, considered a dish of mallows a delicacy, and that such discriminating connoisseurs as the Chinese still use mallows in some of their fine dishes.

These latter references were enough to start me searching for marsh-mallows in order to try their esculent properties. I found them in great plenty (growing in the marshes along the lower reaches of the Delaware River), gathered a supply, and started experimenting. I found that the outer, corky layer easily peeled away, leaving a slender, white, tapering root, about a foot long. Guessing that the fibers would be bothersome if I cooked the roots whole, I cut them crosswise into ¼-inch slices, which I boiled, in just enough water to cover them, for 20 minutes, then drained. These boiled slices were very bland in taste, slightly sweet, mucilaginous, and—let's face it—a bit slimy.

Further processing seemed indicated, so I gently fried the boiled slices in butter, adding some chopped onion for savoriness. When the mallow was lightly browned and the onion was clear and yellow, I judged them done and sat down to my novel lunch of Fried Mallow Roots while it was still piping hot. All sliminess had disappeared, and the onion had contributed exactly the needed flavor. The Romans were right; this is a very palatable vegetable dish.

When I drained the boiled slices of mallow, I saved the water, and now I turned my attention to that. When cold, it was mucilaginous and very viscid, resembling raw egg white. I tried beating it, and it readily whipped into a stiff froth that didn't melt down again in a hurry. This vegetable egg white solved a minor problem for me. I have a friend who is such a strict vegetarian that he won't even eat eggs or gelatin. I had long wanted him to taste some of my wild-fruit chiffon pies, but since they contain both eggs and gelatin he wouldn't touch them. I knew I could substitute Irish moss for the gelatin, but until now, I had not found a vegetable substitute for egg whites.

I make chiffon pies of almost any wild fruit that is available, but it was late August when I made these experiments with mallow, and May-apples, *Podophyllum peltatum*, were ripening in every nook and hollow, and there is simply no better chiffon-pie timber than ripe May-apples. I made a graham-cracker crust and set it aside to cool. On a trip to the seashore I had gathered a quantity of Irish moss, and after washing it through several fresh waters, had put it to dry in my attic. It had dried into a hard, horny substance that didn't look at all promising as food. However, a handful of this stiff, dried seaweed was put to soak in cold water, and in a few minutes it was completely reconstituted, looking as if it had just been pulled from its native rocks.

The bloom and stem ends were cut away from 1 pound of May-apples, which were then quartered, and the pieces were put in a small saucepan with 1 cup of water and 1 cup of sugar. I then tied ¼ cup of the soaked Irish moss in a little square of cheesecloth and submerged it in the cooking water. The fruit was barely simmered for 20 minutes. I stirred it occasionally, always being sure that the seaweed bag was submerged at the end of each stirring. When the pot was removed from the heat, I lifted out the bag of Irish moss, squeezed it against the side of the vessel with a spoon to remove as much glutinous matter as possible, then discarded it, cloth and all. Fruit and liquid were put through a food mill to remove the seeds and skins from the May-apples, and the resulting semiliquid mixture was put aside to cool and coagulate.

I didn't want it to set too hard before incorporating it with the beaten mallow extract, so as soon as it thickened slightly, I put nearly a cupful of the viscid mallow-water in a large mixing bowl and beat it with the electric mixer until it stood in very stiff peaks. When the May-apple mixture had set just until it would mound slightly when spooned, I gave it a good beating with the electric mixer and then folded the two together, gently but thoroughly, and spooned this immediately into the graham-cracker crust. The filling was generous, but it was stiff enough to stand in high peaks, so I piled up a pie a mile high with a fancy swirl on top. When this had chilled in the refrigerator until firmly set I bore it in triumph to my vegetarian friend.

Despite its great height, the pie cut easily and cleanly, and when transferred to a plate, each piece held its shape perfectly. It was light as a pleasant thought, and, since both Irish moss and mallow are very bland, the hauntingly delicious May-apple completely dominated the flavor. Some day I will find a wild-plant product that will make a good piecrust, and when that happens I am going to substitute home-made maple sugar or wild honey for the sugar in the above recipe and create a perfect pie for which every ingredient is foraged from the wild. Such a project will not only make a good pie, but will also do something magnificent for the soul of the cook.

Mallow has been used as a medicinal herb since before the dawn of history and still finds an honored place in most pharmacopoeias of the world. It is no wonder drug with magic healing properties, but it is a dependable demulcent and emollient, with no astringency and no bad taste. Because of its soothing, softening, protective, coating qualities it has been found useful in inflammation and irritation of the respiratory tract, urinary passages, and alimentary canal, and in ointments and poultices for external sores and irritations. It was once thought to be a prime prophylactic against all sorts of illnesses, and Pliny writes, "Whosoever shall take a spoonful of the Mallows, shall that day be free of all diseases that may come to him." If this were only true it would certainly be a simple method of maintaining health and avoiding sickness. I think I'll try this with "an apple a day" for double insurance.

The most commonly used home remedy made of this plant is Mallow Water. In the old herbals there are any number of recipes for making this decoction, but I find that the water that is poured off marsh-mallow roots that I prepare for food serves excellently. If you must use dried marsh-mallow roots (they can be bought from most druggists) shave 3 ounces of the root into 3 cups of water, boil it down until only 2 cups are left, then strain.

At our house we mix this viscid liquid with honey and orange juice, equal parts of each, and take it freely, a tablespoonful at a time, for coughs, minor irritations of the throat, or bronchitis. A wineglassful will act as a very gentle laxative. Its efficacy in this area is no doubt due to its demulcent and lubricative qualities, and not to any drug action. This syrup is smooth, palatable, nutritious, completely free of any dangerous or drastic drugs, and can safely be given to children.

The leaves and flowers of marsh-mallow have the same properties as the root, and 3 ounces of either the dried leaves or the dried flowers can be substituted for the dried root in the above recipe. Gather the leaves or flowers on a dry day, after the sun has dried off the dew, spread them on papers in a warm room, and let them dry until friable. Crumble and store in tightly closed containers until used.

Externally, warm poultices of either the leaves or the crushed root of marsh-mallow have long been trusted domestic remedies for wounds that have developed what was then called "blood poisoning," or "mortification," old-fashioned terms for infection, and the beginning stages of gangrene. Its efficacy in clearing up these infections has earned marsh-mallow the alternate common name of "mortification root." When I was a small boy running barefoot, I cut my foot on a rusty hoe blade and developed a bad infection, with ugly, lurid streaks radiating from the wound up my leg, while the whole leg and the gland in my groin were throbbing with pain. My mother diagnosed blood poisoning, put me to bed, and bound to the wound a great, mushy poultice of mallow leaves and shaved slippery-elm bark. She applied this damp mass as hot as I could stand it and then added a hot-water bottle to keep it warm. She renewed it, using new materials whenever it became cold, and by the next day the throbbing pain was gone, the swelling was down, the red streaks had disappeared, and the wound was healing nicely.

Years later I was skin diving in Hawaii when a wave dashed me against a reef, cutting my arm slightly on the sharp coral. The wound was so minor that I forgot to care for it, and a few days later there were those same ugly red streaks radiating from the puncture and the gland in my armpit was swollen and very sensitive. Neither mallow nor slippery elm was available, but an old Hawaiian woman made a slimy poultice of mashed skins of very ripe bananas, which also have emollient properties, and bound it to my arm as hot as I could endure it. Incongruously, she covered this primitive poultice with a modern electric hot pad to keep it warm. Again, within 24 hours the pain was gone, all infection had disappeared, and the wound was getting well.

In trying to understand the rationale of this treatment, and how such widely different substances could have identical effects, I came to the conclusion that any emollient plant substance would do as well. I reasoned that the poultice material merely softened the wound and kept it open while the heat did the work. However, when I recently learned, from an unimpeachable source,* that the skins of ripe bananas actually have a powerful antibiotic action that is effective against both fungal and bacterial infections, I began to revise my beliefs. Maybe mallow and slippery elm also have in them antibiotic substances that actually destroy the organisms responsible for infections. The "old wives" seem to have been using antibiotics empirically and intuitively, long before the medical profession developed them as we know them now. I would like to recommend both mallow and slippery elm as promising sources to those who are engaged in searching for antibiotics among higher plants.

Those who live where the marsh-mallow does not grow need not be deprived of its benign qualities, for this good plant comes from a good family, the malvaceae, and has about a thousand relatives, widely distributed and many of them exceedingly abundant. All members of this prominent plant family contain the mucilaginous, demulcent, emollient properties of the marsh-mallow; none of them are poisonous, acrid, or even bitter, and a great many of them are either actively or potentially useful to man in more ways than one. Among ornamentals the flamboyant hibiscus, the lordly hollyhock, and the friendly rose-of-Sharon all claim kinship with the marsh-mallow. Cotton, by far the most important fiber plant of the world, is a member of this family, and okra, an important food plant of southern United States and Africa, also belong in this group. Even more important, from our point of view, is the dwarf mallow, *Malva rotundifolia*, which grows wild along roadsides, about farmyards, and in cultivated ground over most of this country.

* "Antibiotics That Come From Higher Plants," by Schaffer, Scott, and Fontaine, 1950–1951 Yearbook of Agriculture, U.S. Department of Agriculture.

Dwarf mallow, also called cheese mallow, fairy cheeses, or doll cheeses, is an immigrant from Europe that has become thoroughly naturalized and is now so common and inconspicuous that it is likely to be overlooked. It is a low herb that springs up in any ground that has been disturbed; though the stems may be as much as two feet long they tend to lie across the ground, and the whole herb seldom rises more than eight inches high. The leaves are rounded heart-shape, from one to two inches in width, and the same in length, dark-green, with the margins wavy and edged with rounded teeth, and the leafstalks are very long for so small a plant. From the axils of these long leafstalks spring several flowers, too small to be conspicuous, but quite pretty when examined closely. They are five-petaled, with a form like a tiny hibiscus that failed to get completely open, pale lavender in color, with darker lavender stripes running lengthwise on each petal. These flowers soon fall and are followed by round, flat fruits, about one-fourth inch across, with scalloped edges, the whole fruit tightly wrapped in the five-parted green calyx. The plant is everbearing, having flowers, fruit, and dried seeds on the same plant from June until frost.

I suppose my mother first taught me how to remove the green calyx and eat the little greenish-white mallow fruits, but this must have been during the period of infantile amnesia. From as early as I can remember, these tiny "cheeses," or "biscuits," were staple fare at the camps I pitched out in the "Wild West," which was the weed-grown vacant lot next door. This was probably the first wild food I ever ate, and the fact that I could provide my own real and edible provisions was immensely satisfying. How do they taste? I'm afraid I can't be objective about that, for to me the flavor is blended with pokeberry war paint, Indian camps, and the age of six, and these are very pleasant fare for a middle-aged man to chew on, now. I never considered these little fruits delicious, and I doubt that I ever called them good. They taste slightly herby, very bland and mucilaginous, but they have no bad or bitter taste, and I found them very acceptable austerity rations for the little explorer and Indian fighter who set up his camp among the high sunflowers, far from civilization. If it weren't for the sentimentality and nostalgia their flavor excites, I would have to admit that mallow fruits taste very much like nothing at all to the spoiled taste buds that I now possess.

Recently I wondered if I could make Mallow Water of dwarf mal-

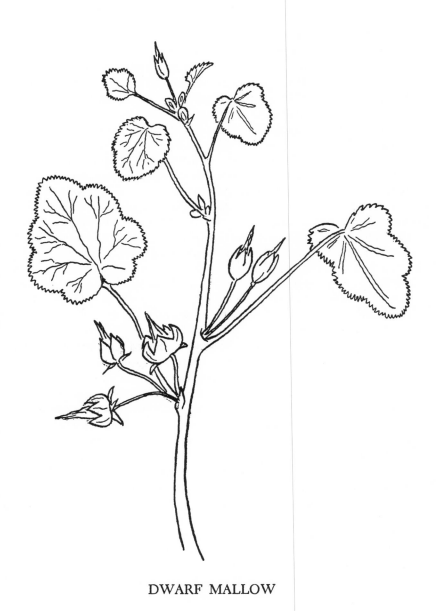

DWARF MALLOW

low. The roots were long and thin as knitting needles, and it took quite a few of them to make a cupful of cleaned, chopped root. When this was boiled as directed for marsh-mallow root, the drained-off water was thin and not nearly as mucilaginous as when real marsh-mallow was used. The boiled roots were tough and fibrous and were not tempting as food.

Next I tried using the tiny fruits I had eaten as a child. At first I removed these fruits from the thin calices that surrounded them, but this proved to be a very tedious operation, and I later discovered it was entirely unnecessary, for these green husks become tender when cooked, taste good, and probably contribute to the yield of mucilage. This discovery speeded up the picking job considerably. A cupful of these little fruits, boiled in 2 cupfuls of water until the juice was reduced to 1 cupful, yielded a viscid Mallow Water that seemed almost identical to that prepared from marsh-mallow roots. It would even whip into a stiff froth, like egg whites, and I found I could use this liquid in any preparation that called for Mallow Water. After draining, the boiled "cheeses" were edible when merely salted, and when fried with onions they were nearly the equal of the Fried Mallow Roots described earlier.

During these experiments I became impressed with the emollient action of mallow. When I rubbed Mallow Water into my hands it made the skin soft and supple, suggesting that an excellent Mallow Hand Lotion could be made from this decoction. My first experiment was a ridiculous failure. I reasoned that a mixture of several emollient substances would produce a truly superior product, so I boiled 1 ounce of Irish moss in 2 cups of water for 10 minutes, strained it, and to this liquid added 1 cup Mallow Water, 2 ounces glycerin, and the juice of 1 lemon, and poured it all into a narrow-necked bottle. This was my first mistake, for I had not foreseen that the Irish moss would make my lotion into a jelly too stiff to be poured from such a bottle. In order even to try my lotion I had to set the bottle in hot water until the jelly remelted, then transfer it to a wide-mouthed container. Although it promptly jelled again, it was a semiliquid jelly that easily melted on the skin, and it seemed an excellent lotion, or cream, to cure and prevent winter chap and dishpan hands. My wife thought it as good as any hand lotion she had ever used. However, we enjoyed it only a few days, for it soon became obvious that this jelly was an excellent culture medium, and long whiskers of gray-green mold appeared in the jar. I threw it out and made a fresh batch, but this time I heated the freshly made lotion to almost boiling, then added 3 ounces of pure grain alcohol, and quickly poured the liquid into sterilized baby-food jars and sealed them. We opened one jar at a time, as needed, and no mold grew in the jar in use. We had a fine hand lotion that seemed to us to be superior to any we could buy.

Later I discovered another use for this Mallow Hand Lotion. One night I was being kept awake by a nervous, unproductive cough that sometimes plagues me, so I went to the jam cupboard to get some violet syrup, which usually relieves such a cough for me. I couldn't find the bottle of violet syrup, but my eyes fell on the little jars of hand lotion. In my mind, I quickly ran through the list of ingredients: Irish moss, mallow, glycerin, lemon juice, alcohol—nothing harmful there, and all likely ingredients for a cough medicine. I opened a jar and took a spoonful. It wasn't delicious, but I have tasted worse medicines, and its emollient properties did soothe my throat and banish my cough. A combination hand lotion and cough syrup! How's that for a versatile medicine? When I went back to bed, I mentioned to my wife that I couldn't find the violet syrup. She said, "Why don't you take a spoonful of that borage-blossom jam? I've found that will relieve a cough." I answered, "I don't need to; I've just cured it by taking a dose of hand lotion."

31. Listen to the Basswood Tree

(*Tilia americana*)

ONE DAY in late spring, a little Pennsylvania Dutch boy and I were making our way along a brushy stream looking for a good fishing hole. When we stopped for a breather, my small companion suddenly cocked his ear and said, "I hear a basswood tree." This statement simply didn't make sense to me. I had not been aware that the basswood was capable of making any kind of sound, let alone one that was distinctive enough so that the species could be recognized by sound alone. For a moment I wondered whether he had heard the tree give a cry of pain, or had detected a mother basswood clucking to her young. The little boy now brought another of his senses into play. He tilted his nose into the air and began sniffing the warm breeze, moving about as he sniffed. Finally he said, "I smell it over this way," and plunged into the brush.

Hunting trees by sound and smell was something new to me, but I followed, and after a few yards of heavy brush near the stream we came into an opening, in the center of which stood a noble basswood, about a hundred feet high. The tree was covered with hundreds of pounds of creamy-white blossoms that were perfuming the whole neighborhood. Wild honeybees had gathered by tens of thousands to harvest the copious flow of nectar, and, incidentally, to pollenize the flowers so that the basswood would be able to bear fruit. The combined buzzing of those thousands of wings made a deep humming sound of such volume that it could be heard for several hundred yards. The mystery was solved. What my little friend had heard had been neither a cry of pain nor a mother's clucking; it was the basswood's mating call!

The American basswood is a close relative of the European linden, so often planted in this country as an ornamental or shade tree, and the two trees have identical uses. The chief difference between them is that the American species has much larger leaves. The Old World linden has leaves that are two to four inches long, and those of its American counterpart are four to six inches long. On both, the leaves are of a somewhat lopsided heart-shape, dark-green above and lighter below, edged with sharp serrations. The flowers, borne in flat clusters, are creamy-white and very fragrant, and each flower has five petals and five sepals. These are followed in a remarkably short while by green, spherical fruits about a quarter-inch in diameter, the first fruits achieving full size before the last of the blossoms fall. The wood is white, close-grained, soft, and very tractable, making it a favorite with wood-carvers and makers of woodcuts.

Basswood and linden are some of the finest honey plants in existence, and the honey the bees make from this fragrant nectar is reputed to be the best-flavored and most valuable honey in the world. It seldom appears on the market for general use, as it is quickly bought up for use in medicine and fine liqueurs. On a few occasions, while robbing a bee tree in the forest, I have found a few combs of pure basswood honey, and it is, indeed, a rare treasure.

The use of the dried flowers of linden and basswood for making a tea-like hot drink is widespread. The French enjoy a number of herbal "tisanes," and that made from linden blossoms is one of their favorites. Several writers report that most French households, at least formerly, kept a supply of these dried blossoms on hand, and this *tilleul* can even be ordered in some French restaurants. Gather the blossoms when they are full-blown and spread them on papers in a warm room. When they are fully dry, pack them in tightly covered containers. Make the tea exactly as you would Oriental tea. This hot infusion is the only herbal medicine made of the linden and basswood, and it is well worth drinking for pleasure alone. Medicinally, it is reported to be calmative and restorative, being given as a home remedy for nervousness, hysteria, insomnia, and cramps. One reference says, "If the flowers used for making the tisane are too old they may produce symptoms of narcotic intoxication." I don't believe this.

I have made tea from flowers of all ages, from unopened buds to those that have already fallen from the tree, and have also eaten these blossoms in greater quantities than anyone would ever use in making tea, and have never suffered even the slightest symptom of any untoward effect. If it is narcosis or kicks you are seeking, look elsewhere, for linden or basswood blossoms will never furnish them.

If basswood or linden blossoms are steeped in the bath water, or a quantity of the tea is added to a long, leisurely, hot bath, it is supposed to allay nervousness and promote sleep. The best way to do this is to stuff an odd sock with either the fresh or dried blossoms and tie it on the bathtub spigot so the hot water running through the flowers can dissolve out their fragrance. I tried this and fairly reveled in the luxury of it, feeling like a Roman aristocrat in his perfumed bath.

If basswood had no other uses than those already outlined, it would be a tree worth knowing, but imagine my excitement when I ran across an article which stated that the sap of lindens and basswoods contained considerable sugar and could be used, like that of the sugar maple, to make syrup and sugar. Even more exciting was the statement that if the flowers and fruit, which appear on the tree at the same time, were ground fine, the resulting paste would "perfectly" resemble chocolate in taste. It was stated that there had been an attempt to develop this "chocolate" commercially in Germany during the time of Frederick the Great, and that the experiments had been abandoned only when it was found that the "chocolate," while perfectly good when fresh, would not keep very well. The writer thought that with modern knowledge and techniques this difficulty might easily be overcome and suggested that here was a great opportunity for some enterprising Yankee.

I was determined to be that Yankee, even though "Yankee" is not a kind word where I was born and spent my early years. I first read these words in winter, and I could hardly wait until spring to make up a supply of this linden sugar and linden chocolate. In fact I didn't wait until spring to try the sugar-making. During the January thaw I usually tap a few maples for some early syrup, for this time often brings a spell of good maple-sugaring weather to my area of Pennsylvania, a full two months before it is experienced farther north. I had both European lindens and American basswoods available, and put a few taps in each kind as I was tapping the maples. The maples fairly gushed sap, but not a single drop flowed from the lindens or basswoods. Hanging a bucket on these spiles (spouts) was simply a waste of time. Later, during the regular maple-sugaring season, I again tried tapping these trees. Same result. I kept tapping linden and basswood trees into late spring, until the leaves appeared, and I have yet to collect my first drop of sap from either of them. Maybe they require an entirely different tapping method. It might be that if one cut a series of grooves through the bark and cambium, in an ascending herringbone pattern, somewhat as a rubber tree is tapped, some sap could be induced to flow, but I have never felt at liberty to disfigure such a beautiful tree in this fashion. Mark this attempt down as a total failure.

I consoled myself with the thought that I would soon be able to manufacture my own chocolate. As soon as the first of the almost instant fruits appeared I gathered a supply, mixed them with some of the flowers, and ground it all to a smooth paste. It turned a light-brown color and didn't look at all like chocolate, and when I tasted it I found that its resemblance to chocolate didn't live up that "perfectly" at all. I don't know what kind of chocolate Europeans had at the time of Frederick the Great, but this paste certainly didn't taste like any chocolate that I am accustomed to eating. Actually, I don't think I would have even been reminded of chocolate when I tasted it, if it hadn't been suggested by that article I read. It wasn't bad in flavor; when some sugar was added, some might have called it good, but it wasn't chocolate.

I continued experimenting with this food, varying the amounts of fruits and flowers until I discovered that the Basswood Paste I liked best was made of all flowers and no fruits. The ideal instrument for reducing these flowers to a smooth paste is an electric blender. The best concoction using these flowers that I have been able to evolve so far is made as follows: Put 2 cups, tightly packed, of linden or basswood flowers in your blender. Soak 2 tablespoons of unflavored gelatin in ¼ cup of cold water until it is softened, then add 1 cup of boiling water and stir until the gelatin is dissolved. Add 2 cups sugar and stir until this is dissolved. Pour the warm syrup over the basswood blossoms in the blender and blend at high speed until the whole mess is reduced to a very smooth paste. Pour into a square pan and set in the refrigerator overnight. Next day, cut the stiff jelly into cubes, roll each piece in granulated sugar, and it is ready to eat. This candy will keep in the refrigerator for a week or more, but if you wish to keep it longer, spread the pieces on a cookie tin, and place in your freezer until the cubes are hard and solid; then they can be transferred to a freezer container or plastic bag and will keep in your freezer for a year. This is a fairly palatable confection, and when eating it you are undoubtedly getting all those famous medicinal benefits—quelling your hysteria, relaxing your cramps, and dispelling your insomnia. If you have an outstanding imagination you can even fancy that it tastes a bit like chocolate.

Finding that I could eat a considerable quantity of this candy with no ill effects removed all fear of eating the fresh blossoms and fruits directly from the tree. This could be a valuable survival technique in an emergency. While these fruits and flowers are not outstandingly palatable, I have eaten worse things at some dining tables, and I'm sure a really hungry man would appreciate them. They could mean the difference between life and death for a man lost in a forest or for a flier forced down in a remote area. They would fill his stomach, give him energy, and might even allay the nervousness that he would be sure to feel about whether he will ever get out again. I have tried adding these fragrant blossoms to a tossed salad with excellent results. When tempered with an oil-and-vinegar dressing they are really good. Although the linden and basswood have handed me some disappointments, they have also given me a few delightful products. I like these trees.

32. Jewelweed or Wild Touch-me-not

(*Impatiens capensis*)

I HAVE mentioned jewelweed in a previous book, but only as a first-aid measure to prevent ivy poisoning, and it is too interesting a plant to be so lightly dismissed. It is a tender, succulent, tall-growing annual, and is often found in extensive patches in damp woods. It has a tremendous range, being found from Nova Scotia to southern Alaska and south to Florida and Oregon. Jewelweed will sometimes reach a height of four feet under favorable growing conditions, but even at this height it does not become coarse or tough. The tender, fragile, much-branching stems are light-green in color, very juicy, and strangely, this juice is a light-orange color when expressed. The leaves, from minute to about three inches long, are egg-shaped with a point at the outer end and widespread serrations on the margins. The common name, jewelweed, was given this plant because its leaves are unwettable—that is, rain will stand on the leaves, in round drops shining like jewels, without ever wetting the leaf surface.

The jewelweed bears pretty flowers, butter-yellow in color, and these are followed by slipper-shaped seedpods about three-fourths inch long. If these seedpods are touched when they are ripe, they will suddenly split, the two sides curling back into tight spirals with an audible snap, throwing the seeds over the surrounding terrain. It is this habit that gives the plant the common name of wild touch-me-not, or, in some sections, snapweed. I have walked through patches of jewelweed where my passing caused this plainly audible

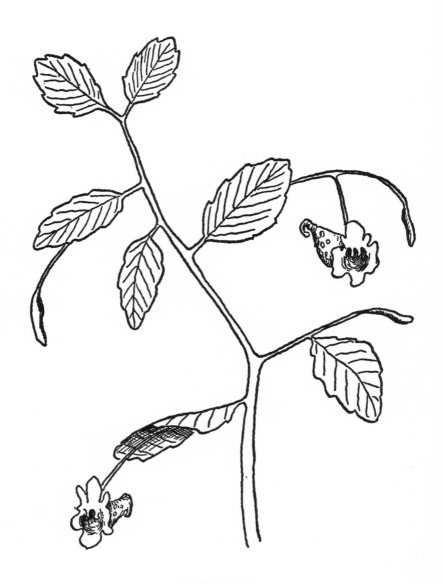

JEWELWEED

snapping sound to come from every plant against which I brushed.

Those who write on wild food are about evenly divided on jewelweed, half of them claiming it is one of the best wild vegetables to be found, and the other half warning that it is poisonous. This is not at all an unusual situation in the wild-food field. Since the publication of my first book on wild foods, I have received dozens of letters taking me to task for recommending for food some plant that "everyone" knows is poisonous. It is seldom twice that the same plant is damned, and if I heeded all these dire warnings there would hardly be a plant left in the wilds that I would dare to eat. I have been warned against May-apples, black-haws, ground-cherries, sumach, wild cherries, elderberries, and only recently I received a letter from a man who said that his neighbor had told him that both persimmons and acorns were deadly poisonous. These stories are not circulated from malice, but from ignorance. A mother doesn't want to risk having her child sample a plant with which she is unfamiliar, so she scares him away from it by telling him it is poisonous. The child grows up and tells his own children and neighbors that this fruit or vegetable is poisonous, for, naturally, mothers don't lie, and so the error spreads.

After reading all the pros and cons I could find about jewelweed, I gingerly experimented with eating it. I gathered the young sprouts in the spring when they were no more than four to six inches high, cut the tender stems into short lengths, and cooked them like green beans, draining away the cooking water. These were seasoned with butter, salt, and a little black pepper, and they were delicious. Later I tried Jewelweed Sprouts in cream sauce, on toast, and they were even better, rivaling asparagus in palatability, although far different in flavor. I suffered not the slightest ill effects from my strange fare, but since the stories of its poisonous nature were so widespread, and emanated from such respectable sources, I decided not to include jewelweed in my first book on wild foods.

Shortly after the book was published, I received a letter from a doctor in Maine, berating me for omitting his favorite wild vegetable, jewelweed. He wrote that he and his family enjoyed jewelweed every spring, considering it one of the finest foods to be found in the wild. His cooking methods were similar to mine. I decided that the word of an M.D. who had experience in eating this plant was better evidence than all the "it is reported to be" references I found in the books, so I have continued to enjoy jewelweed and feed it to my family and guests each spring. No one under my observation has ever suffered even the slightest toxic symptoms.

This does not rule out the possibility that jewelweed might be harmful to certain rare individuals. Allergies and food idiosyncrasies being what they are, this same thing can be said of almost any plant, wild or domestic, that is used as food by man. One reference warned that it might be laxative to some people, but again, the same can be said of most garden vegetables, especially if one eats large amounts of a fresh food after being a long time without it. From my own experience, I would say that jewelweed is an excellent and most palatable vegetable that seems to be perfectly wholesome when eaten in reasonable quantities.

As a medicinal herb, jewelweed is chiefly noted as an emergency prophylactic against ivy poisoning. A great many believe that if one has accidentally brushed against poison ivy, rubbing the exposed part with fresh jewelweed that has first been crushed in the hands will keep any rash from developing. Since jewelweed and poison ivy extend over almost exactly the same range and have identical soil and moisture requirements, the two plants are often found growing together, or at least near one another. I once thought that any beneficent effect of the jewelweed treatment was due to the moisture in this juicy plant, and that one was merely washing away the poisons, but it now appears that this plant actually has some medicinal property that is antagonistic to the poisons in poison ivy. I have heard of several summer camps where the person in charge of first aid boiled down large quantities of jewelweed and used this concentrated juice not only to wash exposed parts to prevent the development of ivy poisoning, but to treat the rash after it had already developed. Several of the poison ivy lotions sold commercially for the treatment of poison ivy rash are really extracts of this plant. I am almost never troubled by poison ivy, but when an untried city guest insists on accompanying me on my jaunts through woods infested with poison ivy, I gather a pound or so of jewelweed, boil it awhile, then suggest that this guest later take a bath, adding the cooking water from the jewelweed to his bath water. Not one guest who has followed this procedure has ever developed poison ivy rash, although many have been heavily exposed to the ivy before bathing.

I tried making some poison ivy lotion similar to that sold commercially with very indifferent success. When a potful of jewelweed was covered with water and boiled down until the liquid was about half of its original volume, the strained juice seemed to be effective both in preventing the rash after exposure to poison ivy and in treating the rash after it had developed. However, the stuff wouldn't keep. Even when kept in the refrigerator it developed strange-looking hemispheres of mold after a few weeks. I tried adding alcohol, and this did seem to preserve it, but a trusting friend who let me apply this lotion to a bad case of ivy poisoning found it very irritating.

Then another friend discovered the secret for which I was searching. He had hired several men to help him clear a brushy lot that was heavily infested with poison ivy, and he was expecting trouble. Before starting the job, he boiled down a quantity of jewelweed to make the kind of watery extract I also manufacture, and because he didn't want to have to boil a new batch every day, he strained the juice into ice trays and froze it in his refrigerator. The answer was so simple that it had escaped me. When it was needed either as a preventive or for treatment, the affected area was simply rubbed with one of these medicated ice cubes, or the cube was allowed to melt and the liquid was applied. The only man on the job who developed ivy poisoning was one who thought all herbal remedies were nonsense and refused to take any precautions. A painful case of ivy poisoning soon caused him to relent, and the rash rapidly cleared up when he began using frozen jewelweed extract.

Since learning this, I have gathered a quantity of jewelweed every spring, boiled it down, and frozen the juice. After being frozen, the cubes can be transferred to a plastic bag and stored in the freezer, so I now have an emergency treatment for poison ivy always available. This has proved very handy, as I seem to get poison ivy only from cleaning out fencerows and flower beds in late fall and early spring when fresh jewelweed is unobtainable.

The early settlers learned from the Indians to use jewelweed, not only in curing and preventing poison ivy rash, but also in treating itch, unhealthy scalp, athlete's foot, and many kinds of dermatitis that we now know are fungal in origin. These uses of jewelweed have long been neglected, even by herbalists and users of home remedies, but it is now proved that jewelweed is a perfectly reasonable and effective treatment for these conditions. The following paragraph is taken from *Crops in Peace and War*, which is the 1950–1951 Yearbook of Agriculture, published by the U.S. Department of Agriculture. This quotation is from an article in the book called "Antibiotics That Come From Higher Plants," written by P. S. Schaffer, William E. Scott, and Thomas D. Fontaine:

"At the University of Vermont, Thomas Sproston, Jr., and associates tested 73 plant extracts, directing particular attention toward those that show fungicidal or fungistatic properties. The most active antifungal extracts were obtained from *Impatiens* (wild touch-me-not), *Cucumis melo* L. (muskmelon), and *Tropaeoleum majus* L. (nasturtium). The crystalline antifungal agent isolated from *Impatiens* was 2-methoxy-1, 4-naphthoquinone."

I'll bet those ancient Indians didn't know, when they put some boiled-down juice of jewelweed on an itchy spot, that they were really treating a fungal disorder with a superscientific fungicide called 2-methoxy-1, 4-naphthoquinone. Neither did I until I read this article. To test the fungicidal properties of this plant, the experimenters used a watery extract of the plant similar to the one I recommend for treating poison ivy. It was only after determining that this liquid had fungicidal properties that the crystalline agent responsible for these benign effects was isolated and extracted. I have not had the itch, unhealthy scalp, athlete's foot, or any kind of fungoidal dermatitis, since reading the above, but I see no reason why frequent applications of that plain, boiled-down, cooking water from jewelweed, or the ice cubes made of it, would not be an effective treatment for these disorders. Jewelweed seems a good plant to know.

33. Medicinal Christmas Decoration:

MISTLETOE AND HOLLY

CHRISTMAS TREE lights have no magic unless they are reflected in the eyes of children. The old farmhouse that is our home tries to be gay in its holiday dress, but the sense of wonder, so characteristic of little ones and so essental to Christmas, is not here. The spontaneous "Oh!" escaping from round little mouths under widened, shining eyes, is missing, and I like to have an "Oh!" in things at Christmas. My sons and grandchildren are all far away this year, and today I miss them. We are not unhappy, for this has been a very rewarding year, with no family disasters to mar it. My wife and I exchanged presents this morning that were made far more precious by the tried and tested love that went with them. There will be plenty of quiet joy and contentment in this house today, but, still, I am tempted to call one of my younger and more prolific neighbors to ask if I can borrow a child or two, just for today.

I resolved I would not touch a typewriter on Christmas Day, but the sheer childlessness of this day has driven me back to my natural children, the herbs, fruits, roots, seeds, and foliage with which nature fills my life so wonderfully. It is dark and rainy outside, so I stay indoors studying the wreaths and sprays around me, and meditate on mistletoe and holly.

MISTLETOE
(*Phoradendron flavescens*)

American mistletoe, while in the same family of plants as European mistletoe, *Viscum album*, is far from being identical with it, and the two plants have quite different medicinal properties. American mistletoe, according to a textbook on pharmacology, acts as a powerful stimulant to smooth muscles, producing a rise in blood pressure and increasing the contraction of the intestines and uterus. It has been recommended as a circulatory and uterine stimulant. On the other hand, European mistletoe is said to reduce blood pressure and have an antispasmodic effect in small doses, although overdoses have been reported to cause spasms. So we see that in some ways these two closely related plants have almost directly opposite effects on the human system. This illustrates the danger of trying to apply European herbal writings to related, but different, species in America. Even closely related plants can sometimes have dramatically different effects when used in home remedies.

There is no need to describe American mistletoe. If you are not already familiar with this plant, just look up the next time you are unexpectedly kissed during the winter holidays and study the little plant you are certain to see hanging above you. Only yesterday I was explaining to a sweet old lady that mistletoe could cause a rise in blood pressure, and she said she knew this to be true because when she was a young girl she had often experienced a rise in blood pressure merely from standing under it. This plant of mysterious powers and privileges grows as an evergreen parasite and is found on deciduous trees from New Jersey to Florida and west to the Great Plains. The translucent white berries are poisonous to human beings, and there are reports that children have died from eating them, although most fruit-eating birds relish mistletoe berries and seem to eat them with impunity. I am often asked whether all berries one sees birds eating are safe for human consumption; mistletoe is a good illustration that bird tastes are not a guide to edibility. Seeing a bird eat a berry only proves that it is safe for birds to eat.

Crush one of these soft berries between your fingers. You will find that the clear pulp is quite sticky and full of tiny seeds. When a bird eats mistletoe berries some of this sticky pulp with its contained seeds is likely to stick to the bird's beak. Birds are cleanly creatures, and sometimes after flying to another limb, or even to another tree, the bird will wipe his beak on the limb on which he is sitting, and the next rain will wash the small seeds down into a crack. This is the way mistletoe spreads itself through the forest. When a seed sprouts, it sends its root through the bark and actually into the wood of its host.

Mistletoe is a true parasite, appropriating as much of the tree's sap as it needs, and it has the power to take this food selectively, so that it does not have to assume the same composition as its host. Mistletoe has been found that contained twice as much potash and five times as much phosphate as its host tree.

Our custom of kissing under mistletoe came from pagan sources. A beautiful but somewhat watered-down version of a Scandinavian legend says that formerly mistletoe was a symbol of hate. Its magic was so potent that it could even overcome the immortality of the gods; Balder, the Scandinavian god of peace, was killed by an arrow of mistletoe wood. A world without peace was unendurable even before the invention of nuclear weapons, so Balder's life was restored at the petition of the other gods and goddesses. To prevent other fatalities among the gods, mistletoe was given into the keeping of the god of love, and it was ordained that everyone passing under it should receive a kiss, to show that this plant had become a symbol of love instead of hate.

In some of the old pagan fertility rites involving mistletoe, the intimacies were even closer than mere kissing. I wonder if there is not an echo of these ancient observances in the fact that many old herbals recommend an infusion of mistletoe as a cure for sterility. Perhaps some of those old pagan rites could cure certain kinds of sterility today.

I know of only one home remedy that can be made of mistletoe, and I consider even its use ill-advised. A friend of mine who comes from the South suffers from low blood pressure, and, when acute, it causes a sort of anxious depression that is very bothersome. Acting on the advice of his herb-wise old grandmother, he takes a cup of hot mistletoe infusion, made by pouring a cup of boiling water over a dozen mistletoe leaves, whenever he begins feeling nervous and depressed. He claims this dispels the mental conditions associated with his trouble and makes him feel better generally. A slight rise in blood pressure could account for the effects he claims to feel, but his is a condition that should be treated by a competent doctor. Modern medicine has scientific remedies for his condition that would probably be safer and more efficacious than mistletoe.

I do not recommend that mistletoe be used in any home remedies, for its medicinal properties are too ill-defined and uncertain in their actions for amateur dosing, and the illnesses for which it is recommended are better treated by a professional doctor. However, let no one thereby conclude that mistletoe is useless; any plant that encourages friendly kissing by people who would not otherwise get an opportunity to kiss one another is far from useless.

Besides the common Christmas mistletoe there are about five other species of *phoradendron* in the United States. The only one of these secondary species with which I am familiar is *P. juniperinum,* which was common on the junipers of New Mexico where I spent the latter part of my boyhood. While it resembles common mistletoe in its parasitic habit of growth, it resembles it not at all in appearance. Probably as an adaptation to the arid region in which it grows, the leaves of this juniper mistletoe have degenerated into mere scales, giving it the appearance of being leafless. It is seen as a cluster of yellow-green, forking stems, quite brittle and easily broken. I know of no medicinal use for it, but it apparently is not harmful to ruminants, as goats are extremely fond of it and I have observed them standing on their hind legs to reach it, or even climbing low trees to eat this delicacy. I have never tried tasting it, but since I spent all my late adolescence in the region where it abounds, I can vouch for the fact that it works just as well for kissing purposes as does the eastern species.

HOLLY
(*Ilex opaca*)

The holly in the wreaths and sprays about me also has some claim to our attention. It was a pagan custom to "deck the halls with bows of holly" during the winter Saturnalia, but early Christians soon saw in the prickly leaves and blood-red berries of the holly wreath a symbol of the crown of thorns that Christ was forced to wear at his crucifixion. This would seem to make holly a more appropriate symbol for Easter, so its use at Christmas was probably an accommodation to carry on the traditional pagan custom. The pagan winter festival of the Saturnalia came about a week before Christmas, and an early edict of the church forbids Christians to decorate their houses with evergreens at the same time as do their pagan neighbors. This was probably the origin of the superstition, still prevalent in England, that it is unlucky to bring holly into the house before Christmas Eve.

The boughs of holly we bring into our houses at Christmas in

America are cut from a native tree, *Ilex opaca,* which grows wild in acid, woodland soils, chiefly near the coast, from Maine to Florida, west to Arkansas and Texas, and again north, up the Mississippi Valley, to Missouri and Indiana. It has also been planted as an ornamental or crop tree in many other areas. It is cultivated in the Pacific Northwest where ample rainfall and a deep acid soil built by generations of giant conifers shedding their needles have created ideal conditions for its growth.

As a medicinal plant, both the berries and the leaves of holly are used. The berries are reported to be a powerful emetic, even small doses causing violent vomiting. This is one herbal medicine I have not tried on myself, nor do I intend to. Some American Indian tribes considered vomiting a cleansing process and took herbs to induce it before certain religious ceremonies, but I find it a very uncomfortable process and will not deliberately induce it in myself, nor do I recommend that you do so. Holly berries are beautiful, but they are not for eating. Again, some birds seem immune to their effects, and any holly berries left over until spring are usually cleaned up by the birds.

It is the leaves of holly that chiefly interest me, for the home remedy made from them is pleasant to take and benign in its effects. These glossy leaves are reported to be diaphoretic, to help reduce fever, and to be tonic in action. They are taken as a hot infusion, or Holly Tea, and one writer says that the poor people of the Black Forest region of Germany have used Holly Tea as a tasty hot beverage purely for pleasure and not for its reputed medicinal benefits. I did try this beverage—in fact, I had a steaming cup of Holly Tea about an hour ago. To make a palatable tea of holly leaves, you must roast them, not only until they are thoroughly dried, but until they are quite brown. They are then crumbled, the larger stems and veins are picked out, and the infusion is made exactly as Oriental tea is made. The crumbled leaves tend to float, so it is necessary to strain the tea before drinking it. Try it with sugar and milk, if you like these additions in your regular tea.

Taking this tea very hot, while one is in bed, will induce sweating, but whether it is more efficient in this respect than plain hot water I cannot judge. It was formerly given in this way for catarrh and pleurisy, and was thought to be effective in lowering fever, stimulating the appetite, and making the patient more comfortable.

It is interesting to note that Paraguay Tea, a favorite drink in

South America, is made of *I. paraguayensis*, a tree closely related to our Christmas holly. Paraguay Tea contains considerable caffeine, and is definitely stimulating, but our Holly Tea is not so fortified and must be consumed for its minor medicinal benefits and its pleasant taste. Now you know what to do with those old holly wreaths after Christmas.

Christmas day is about gone, and fragrant smells arise from the kitchen where our Christmas night dinner is being prepared. I went lunchless, except for one cup of appetite-stimulating holly tea, so that I could work up a ravenous appetite for the feast to come. Through the magic of this typewriter I have brought you into my house as my Christmas guest, and as we have discussed the magic and mystery of holly and mistletoe, my childless loneliness has evaporated. Outside, the clouds have cleared away, and a sunset glow makes the whole countryside warmly beautiful. Thanks to you, it has been a joyful day. Come again.

34. Cleavers or Goosegrass

(Galium Aparine)

DESPITE that terminal "s," cleavers is singular. Cleavers is a weak-stemmed sprawling herb that can't possibly stand upright unless it is climbing on and supported by surrounding vegetation. The thin, quadrangular stem may reach a length of two to five feet and bears on its angles backward-curving bristles that enable it to climb up anything it encounters. Every few inches on this weak stem there is a swollen joint with a whorl of six to eight lance-shaped leaves about a half-inch long and a quarter-inch broad. A botanist has pointed out that this leaf whorl is really only two opposite leaves, and the other apparent leaves are actually *stipules*, or basal appendages to the leaf proper that have evolved into exactly the same shape as the true leaves. In the axils of the real leaves are borne the slender flower stalks, each bearing from one to three star-shaped, greenish-white, inconspicuous little flowers, and these are followed by bristly, two-lobed globular little dry fruits about an eighth of an inch in diameter. The backward-curving bristles on these fruits enable them to cling to anything that brushes against them, a very efficient method of scattering the seeds far and wide.

And far and wide they have been scattered, for this weakly plant is found from Newfoundland to Alaska and south into Mexico, then on around the world in Asia and Europe. Asa Gray, the great American botanist, considered this plant a native of North America, although he did note that cleavers along the East Coast were probably introduced from Europe. It is my opinion, for what it is worth, that this plant was entirely unknown in America before the coming of the white man. I base this belief on anthropological, not botanical,

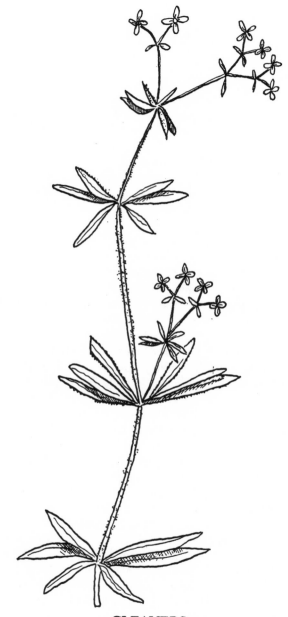

CLEAVERS
(as supported by other vegetation)

evidence. Cleavers has long been recognized in Europe as a valuable medicinal, food, and beverage herb, but the American Indians made no use of it that I can discover. These tribes, with their rich and sophisticated ethnobotany, would surely have discovered a few of the many virtues of cleavers had the plant been around for all the ages that the Indian inhabited this continent before the coming of the white man. The fact that this herb preceded Europeans into the western wilderness and was found behaving like a native when the white man overtook it there proves nothing about a plant as mobile as cleavers. Any Indian, or even any animal, traveling west could have, all unknowingly, carried the sticky little seeds in clothing, hair, or fur, to be dropped in an entirely new area, so the plant could easily have established itself all over North America hundreds of years before very much of this continent was explored.

Though common and abundant over an extremely far-flung area, cleavers are not well known to most laymen. Growing best in damp thickets amidst an abundance of other vegetation, this herb is seldom noticed by the average unobservant hiker unless it is pointed out to him. However, cleavers are about to emerge from their obscurity, for a secret that will bring them undying fame is about to be revealed. According to all the old herbalists this is the reducing diet *par excellence*, painlessly paring pounds from plump persons. There's its slogan, all ready to be woven into neat singing commercials. Cleavers, beware! I foresee a million women worried about weight out beating the country brush, looking for cleavers. It may even appear on drugstore shelves and in supermarkets, but I'll wager that the women who tramp around rural areas looking for their own will lose more weight.

If this secret was once common knowledge, how did it become lost? That one happens to be easy to answer: the plump figure merely came back in style, and women were then hunting herbs that would help them gain weight rather than lose it. By the time that styles had changed again, in their cyclic fashion, and the lean and lank figure was again popular, women had forgotten how to reduce on cleavers.

Springtime must have been reducing time in ancient England, for that is the only time that cleavers are fit to eat. The dish made from it was called "Lenten pottage," and many a woman must have resolved to pare off a few of those extra pounds during Lent, a very efficient arrangement for making her body more attractive to men and helping to save her immortal soul at the same time. In the northern states it is seldom available during Lent, but to be at its best it should be gathered as early as possible. When gathered very young the whole herb, stems and all, will cook perfectly tender in a few minutes. The best way is to put it in a strainer or colander over boiling water and steam it for about 5 minutes. Then it can be eaten hot as a vegetable, chilled as a salad, or quickly cooled, packed into containers and placed in the freezer so milady can reduce any time of the year that the pounds appear.

I seasoned it with butter when I tried it as a hot vegetable and added an oily dressing when I used it as a salad, hoping the reducing powers of the cleavers would counteract the fattening effect of these foods, but I found I could enjoy it for its spinachy taste alone. I even tried serving it in a cream sauce over toast, and found I liked it this way best of all. According to the old herbalists, cleavers should be cooked in mutton broth, with or without oatmeal, when used as a reducing diet that will "keepe them leane and lanke that are apt to grow fatte." One herbalist recommends that cleavers be cooked with nettle tops to make a Lenten pottage, and I like this, for nettles are one of my favorite wild greens.

The usefulness of cleavers is not exhausted by its value in a reducing diet or as a palatable cooked vegetable. The little two-lobed seedlike fruits make the best coffee substitute of almost any plant growing in our range. This time I do not hesitate to use the word "substitute," for cleavers really try to imitate coffee. This may be a family resemblance, for cleavers belong to the *Rubiaceae*, the natural order of plants to which the coffee tree also belongs, so they are at least distant cousins. The little hard fruits, gathered during the summer when they are full-size and roasted in an oven until they are very brown, can be made into a beverage that smells like coffee and even tastes a little like coffee. It contains no caffeine and therefore is not stimulating like its noble relative, but it is fragrant and wholesome and taken without sugar or cream it might help in those reducing diets.

Cleavers has also been considered a medicinal herb of no mean order, its properties being listed as diuretic, tonic, alterative and somewhat laxative. For medicinal purposes, the herb should be gathered in May or June, when in flower, and dried in a warm room. The home remedy is made, as are so many homemade herbal medicines, by pouring a pint of boiling water over 1 ounce of the dried herb. I was pleasantly surprised when I first tasted this Cleavers Tea, for if the seeds of cleavers try to imitate coffee, the leaves attempt to mimic strong Oriental tea. It must be harmless, for I drank a pint at one sitting with no ill effects, but the recommended dosage is a wineglassful two or three times a day. This was formerly a popular spring drink in rural England and was said to purify the blood, which probably means that it has some constituent that makes the average overwintered Englishman feel better.

This plant has been subjected to some chemurgic investigation and was found to contain starch, chlorophyll, and three distinct acids: a kind of tannic acid that has been named galitannic acid, because it was found in *Galium*; citric acid, the same acid that makes lemons valuable; and a peculiar acid that has been named rubichloric acid because it was found in plants of the natural order *Rubiaceae*. Any medicinal value this plant may have is probably due to these acids. The tea has been given as a remedy for colds in the head, and is probably as effective for this purpose as the hot lemonade that is often given. This tea is also said to be a powerful diuretic, stimulating the secretion of urine, and some herbalists have even claimed that it will dissolve kidney stones and gravel in the bladder. Its efficacy as a reducing aid may be due to its diuretic action, for a drug that will cause an increase in the flow of urine beyond its own contained water will often reduce weight by lowering the water content of the body tissues.

Although a reputed aperient, which means a mild laxative, cleavers tea is also given to cure diarrhea. Any efficacy it has in treating this complaint is probably due to the slight astringency that comes from its tannic acid content. A wineglassful of warm Cleavers Tea, taken at bedtime, is said to have a most soothing effect in cases of insomnia, giving quiet, restful sleep. I would be afraid its diuretic effect would interrupt slumber as much as its soporific effect would promote it, but maybe if you sweetened it with honey, for its hygroscopic powers (water-absorbing qualities), this would offset the water-promoting action of the cleavers and allow you to sleep through the night.

Finally, this same tea, cooled and applied to the face with a soft cloth, is supposed to be excellent for sunburn, to remove freckles, and to make the complexion clear and beautiful. This I have not tried, but I pass it on to others where it might have some chance of success.

35. Great Mullein or Velvet Dock

(Verbascum Thapsus)

FEW PLANTS are known by so many common names. Besides the two given in the title, this wide-ranging and well-known plant is also called flannel leaf, beggar's blanket, Adam's flannel, velvet plant, feltwort, bullock's lungwort, clown's lungwort, Cuddy's lungs, tinder plant, rag paper, candlewick plant, witch's candle, hag's taper, torches, Aaron's rod, Jacob's staff, shepherd's club, and Quaker rouge, to name only a few of the names by which it is known in English alone.

Mullein was originally an Old World plant, and was probably first brought to America by some colonial herbalist who knew of its value in alleviating human ills. Mullein found America a congenial place to grow, and quickly escaped from gardens and spread itself over the land. It is now a very common wild plant from far up in Canada to far down in Florida and west to beyond the Rockies. Thus mullein completed its present circumpolar distribution, for it was already a common wild plant throughout the North Temperate Zone in Europe and Asia. With this around-the-world distribution, mullein has long been known to many peoples of many varying cultures, but all of them agree on its values as a healing herb, and it still finds wide use in the domestic remedies of primitive peoples and even in the official preparations of highly civilized countries. It is a common roadside plant in America, and it thrives in pastures, for no grazing animal will eat it, although it has frequently been administered to cattle as a veterinary medicine, an infusion of the leaves being given to treat coughs in cattle.

Mullein is a biennial, and during the first season appears only as a rosette of large leaves, ten to twenty inches long and four to six inches wide, densely covered with a fine white wool that gives the leaves a silvery appearance and a velvety feel. These leaves persist over the winter, and during the second season a solitary, stout, erect flower stalk rises from the center of the rosette, eventually attaining a height of four to eight feet. This flower stalk is usually unbranched, but it does bear leaves. The leaves near the base of the stem are large and numerous, alternately arranged, ten to sixteen inches long and three to four inches broad, stemless, with the lower part of each leaf adhering to the stalk for about a fourth of its length. These leaves become smaller and scantier toward the top of the stalk and finally merge into the thick, densely crowded flower spike, usually about a foot long, with the flowers opening here and there on the spike, not in regular progression from bottom to top as in most spike-borne flowers. Sometimes one finds a mullein plant with the flower spike branched like a candelabrum, and one or two small branches, appearing near the base of the actual flower spike, are not uncommon, but on most plants the flower spike is solitary. The flowers are stalkless, sulfur-yellow in color, and each blossom appears as a little cup about one inch across, formed of five petals united at their bases to form a short tube. This tube is enclosed in a woolly calyx that is deeply cut into five lobes.

The fresh and dried leaves and the fresh flowers are the parts used in home remedies. The leaves are nearly odorless, mucilaginous, and with a slightly bitter taste. Their principal constituents are gum, resin, a little tannin, and a trace of volatile oil. The flowers contain gum, resin, a yellow coloring principle, sugar, some potassium and calcium, and a small amount of a yellow, volatile oil. The odor is peculiar but agreeable, they are mucilaginous, and the taste is sweet.

Throughout its three-continent range, mullein has been used in a great many preparations for a large variety of illnesses, but all these different peoples seem to agree that an infusion of the fresh or dried leaves is a prime remedy for alleviating the distress of bronchial complaints, hacking coughs, and lung troubles. Gather the leaves in July, lay them in a single layer on newspapers in a warm, dry place, such as a well-ventilated attic room, and allow them to dry for two weeks,

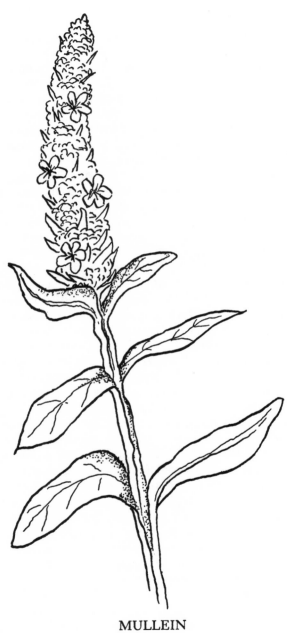

MULLEIN

then crumble and store in a tight container. Since the first-year leaves persist over the winter, the fresh leaves can be gathered any time of the year that they are not covered by snow. The flowers must be gathered fresh while the plant is blooming, usually during July and August. Officially, mullein has been recognized as a valuable demulcent, emollient, expectorant, and mild astringent.

The home remedy made of mullein that is most widely used is an infusion made by boiling 1 ounce of the dried leaves, or 4 ounces of the fresh leaves, in 1 pint of milk for 10 minutes, then straining through a double thickness of muslin. This last is very important, for unless mullein infusions are well-strained through cloth some of the tiny leaf-hairs will remain in the liquid, causing a prickling sensation in the throat. Sweeten the infusion with 1 tablespoon of honey and administer warm, a wineglassful at a time, as needed, the entire amount being taken in one day. I have tried this decoction and find it a pleasant, bland beverage that seems efficacious in relieving a dry, hacking cough. Before tuberculosis was controlled as it is today, this milk infusion of mullein was often given to consumptives, sometimes as much as three pints a day being taken. While this probably never cured the disease, the demulcent, emollient, and expectorant qualities of this benign plant probably did relieve much of the suffering that attends this plague, while the honey and milk furnished healthful nourishment so badly needed by victims of this wasting illness.

Because of its mild astringency, which is due to its tannin content, this same milk infusion has been given as a remedy for diarrhea. Oddly enough, exactly the same remedy has also been given for certain kinds of constipation, its demulcent and lubricative qualities enabling the patient to pass hard stools easily and comfortably. Because of these same qualities, this decoction is said to relieve the pain and irritation of hemorrhoids, if taken regularly.

Dried mullein leaves are sometimes smoked in ordinary tobacco pipes or cigarettes, or the smoke is inhaled from a dish of the burning leaves, for the relief of cough, bronchitis, or asthma. This is the way my Pennsylvania Dutch neighbors most often take mullein, using either dried mullein leaves alone, or mixing them with an equal quantity of the dried leaves of jimson weed, rolling the mixture into cigarettes, and smoking them for the relief of the spasms of asthma.

Part of my boyhood was spent in the Navajo country of New Mexico, and these Indians also know and use mullein. Because of a superficial resemblance between mullein and the tobacco plant, they call mullein "big tobacco." The dried leaves are mixed with ordinary tobacco and smoked for the relief of coughs and bronchial troubles, and the Indians even claim that smoking these mullein cigarettes will correct mild mental disturbances, such as thinking bad thoughts or a tendency to use bad language. (I would like to prescribe these cigarettes for some of our modern novelists.)

Mullein flowers, although they are similar in constitution to the leaves, are used in altogether different ways. The most common use of mullein flowers has been in an ointment made by filling a flat glass flask (you can get one at a drugstore or use an emptied liquor container) with fresh mullein flowers, then covering them with olive oil, and exposing the flask to full sunlight for 21 days. The oil was then strained and stored in a smaller bottle that could be tightly stopped. I tried this process and found that the mullein flowers imparted a deep-yellow color to the olive oil. This mullein oil has found many uses in peasant households in Europe, being used as a local application for frostbite, bruises, and external hemorrhoids, but it was chiefly famous for its reputed ability to cure an earache, a few drops being poured into the affected ear two or three times a day. I have not had an opportunity to try this remedy, but I wish that some competent medical researcher would give it a really comprehensive test and report his results.

A modern source says, "Mullein oil is a valuable destroyer of disease germs. The fresh flowers, steeped for 21 days in olive oil, are said to make an admirable bactericide." * Apparently the ancient herbalists also suspected this power of mullein even though they did not know of the germ origin of infections. They used mullein oil, or applied poultices of mullein leaves to surface infections, and one old herbalist mentions that "Figs do not putrify at all that are wrapped in the leaves of mullein." Since mullein is neither poisonous nor caustic, one suspects that it has no general bactericidal or antiseptic action, and that these accounts indicate the presence of an unsuspected, selective, antibiotic action that might prove extremely useful to medical science if it could be isolated and extracted. I highly recommend mullein to those scientists who are presently searching for useful antibiotics among the higher plants. (See page 212.)

* Maud Grieve, A Modern Herbal (Hafner, 1931).

In England, during the 16th and 17th centuries, there appeared a great rash of irresponsible writing on medicinal herbs. Each self-appointed expert seemed to be trying to outdo all others in the extravagance of the claims made for the healing virtues of every herb mentioned. Reading these old herbals one wonders why they bothered to list so many herbs when, according to their own testimony, any one of them was capable of curing all known ills. Such wild claims had much to do with the disrepute into which herbal medicine later fell, and from which it is only now slowly recovering, as scientists almost apologetically resume the search for healing substances among the botanicals.

As with many other herbs, these old herbals make many irrational claims about the virtues of mullein, and give long lists of most extraordinary cures effected by its use. Some thought that merely carrying a bit of mullein about the person would prevent one's being infected with any illness. A decoction of the root was used to treat such diverse complaints as toothache, cramps, and convulsions. Both the juice of the leaves and the dried, powdered root were reputed to remove warts. The distilled water of the flowers was believed to cure gout. A poultice of the crushed seeds and leaves was used to draw out splinters and thorns that had become imbedded in the flesh. A more logical use was the placing of the thick, woolly leaves inside the stockings to keep the feet warm.

A plant so beneficial as a healing herb was bound to enter deeply into the folklore, magic, and superstitions of the peoples who used it. In ancient England it was believed that those who "trafficked" with the devil used dried mullein stalks, dipped in tallow, to light the orgies of their "witches' sabbaths." In other areas mullein was thought to drive away evil spirits, and in southern Europe, mullein torches were formerly burned at funerals. In India, some considered mullein a sure safeguard against evil spirits and black magic. Even the ancient Greeks considered mullein a powerful agency against evil spirits, and it was this herb that Ulysses carried to protect himself against the wiles of Circe.

When boiling water is poured over fresh mullein flowers it extracts a bright-yellow color that has been used to dye cloth. If dilute sulfuric acid is added to this yellow dye, it will color the cloth a permanent green. By further adding some alkali to the green dye, one obtains a brown color. Thus one can dye cloth three colors using these same flowers. The "drugstore blond" is not nearly as modern as she might like to believe. The beauties of ancient Rome used the yellow dye of mullein flowers to give their hair a golden tint. One ancient authority even claims that a soap made of the ashes of burned mullein leaves, when used as a shampoo, will restore gray hair to its original color. I have not tried this, as I feel that I have earned these gray hairs in honest toil and wear them rather proudly.

Another cosmetic use of mullein gave it the little-used common name "Quaker rouge." Quaker girls considered it immoral to paint their faces, and yet Quaker girls had normal instincts and wanted to appear attractive to the boys. They learned that rubbing a mullein leaf on the cheeks would cause extra blood to flow to that area, giving the cheeks an attractive glow. I tried this, but my complexion is already so florid that it made little difference, so I persuaded a young friend to try it. The second-year leaves from the flower stalk had little effect, but when she rubbed one of the woolly, first-year leaves rapidly over her cheek for a few minutes a rosy hue appeared. Substances that will induce such surface reddening are known as rubefacients, and most of them are quite irritating. It seems likely that it is the irritation of the tiny, woolly hairs of the mullein leaf that causes the reddening. However, in this case, the pretty glow persisted for more than an hour, and my young friend assured me that she felt no discomfort.

Even though you may never intend to use any of the mullein products described in this chapter, let me suggest that the next time you see a tall mullein by the roadside, you stop and really look at it. This plant is so common that we tend to overlook it, or dismiss it as a "mere weed." See how the arrangement of leaves on the tall flower stalk gives the whole plant a graceful symmetry. Examine a leaf closely and see how the dense covering of white hairs gives the leaves a silvery appearance. Feel their velvety smoothness. Observe how the midribs of the leaves adhere to the straight, upright stalk for part of their length, and how the margins of these adherent leaves give the stalk a winged effect. Note the long, curiously wrought flower spike, with dense patches of golden flowers. If you will give all of your attention to a mullein plant for only a few minutes, I am sure you will exclaim, as I have done, "Why, this plant is beautiful!"

36. Curled Dock:

WEED OR FINE FOOD?

(*Rumex crispus*)

A N AGRICULTURAL bulletin begins its description of curled dock, also known as yellow dock, narrow-leaved dock, or common dock, thus, "A troublesome weed very hard to eradicate..." And a writer on wild foods begins his description, "A palatable, easily obtained spring green that is exceedingly wholesome..." It is all in the point of view. Let me try?

Curled dock is a valuable, though generally unappreciated, food and medicinal herb that is common and abundant throughout the United States. Found everywhere on vacant lots, along streams and roadsides, in pastures and waste places, it is a smooth, dark-green plant, one to three feet tall, with a deep-yellow root. A majority of the leaves spring directly from the base. These are six inches to a foot long, one to two inches wide, slenderly lanceolate in shape, rounded at the base, the margins of the leaves being wavy or curly. The flower stalk bears leaves similar in shape to these basal leaves but only about half as large. The flowers are somewhat dry and unattractive, greenish in color, densely arranged in whorls on panicled racemes at the top of the flower stalk. The dry, three-winged fruits that follow the flowers in great abundance turn a rich brown when ripe, making these densely fruiting seedstalks great favorites with those who like to make dried-flower arrangements as autumn decorations.

Dock has long been gathered as a spring green or potherb by those who understand the value and goodness of such food. A quaint old book on home remedies says, "Dock greens should be eaten every

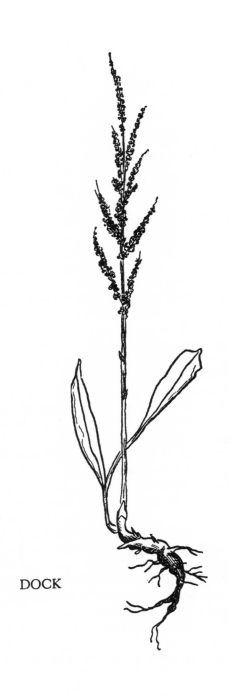

DOCK

spring to thin and purify the blood." I can find no convincing evidence that dock greens ever thin the blood, nor do I find evidence that the blood ever needs thinning, or thickening. "Purifying the blood" is another matter. There are certain toxins and other "impurities" that the body ordinarily eliminates by first combining them with ascorbic acid, which most of us know as vitamin C. In the old days when the winter diet was almost entirely of dried and salted foods, acute vitamin C deficiencies were likely to occur. Then the eating of dock greens with their rich vitamin C content certainly would "purify" the blood and improve the health generally.

In one of the old herbals I find the strange-sounding claim that eating dock greens will tighten loose teeth. This is not the rank superstition it sounds, for the winter diet of those days was often so deficient in vitamin C that advanced cases of scurvy were common by spring. One of the symptoms of scurvy is the loosening of the teeth due to a softening of the gums. Dock greens, being richer in vitamin C than orange juice, did tighten those loose teeth by curing the scurvy, hardening the gums, and improving oral health generally. However, dock greens will not tighten just any loose teeth, but only those that are due to scurvy.

Dock greens are also richer in vitamin A than carrots. I often hear people saying that carrots will brighten the eyes and improve night vision. This is perfectly true if the dullness of the eyes and dimness of night vision is due to a prolonged deficiency of vitamin A. The human body converts carotene, the yellow pigment of carrots, into vitamin A, which is needed to form an essential pigment, rhodopsin, in the retina of the eye. Where vitamin A is deficient in the diet, this pigment cannot form, and the eyes are dull and their ability to adjust to dim light becomes severely limited, but the carrot is not the only vegetable that can cure this condition. There is plenty of carotene in most green, leafy vegetables, where its color is masked by the chlorophyll, and dock is especially rich in this yellow pigment, containing approximately four times as much carotene as carrots. If carrots will brighten your eyes and improve your night vision, dock greens should make them four times as bright and enable you to see in the dark like a cat.

The fact that dock greens are an exceeding healthful vegetable is, I believe, well established, but rather than say, "Dock should be eaten because it is good for you," I would say, "Dock should be eaten because it is good." I seem to notice a direct correlation between palatability and vitamin content in plants used as cooked greens. The higher the vitamin content, the better the taste. In comparing dock to most other greens, wild or domestic, I would say that dock tastes better because it is better; it is as simple as that.

It is enough to make one weep to realize that a great deal of that wintertime scurvy from which many people formerly suffered was totally unnecessary in most localities. Dock refuses to stop growing merely because the weather gets cold. After the first freeze or two, dock often sprouts a whole new crop of tender leaves during Indian summer, and will continue to put up new leaves during any warm spell in winter. In the United States, fresh palatable dock greens can usually be picked, from Philadelphia southward, any time they are not covered with snow.

I am writing these words in central Pennsylvania, on the twenty-first of December, the shortest day of the year. There are scattered patches of snow about, and already there have been several nights when the mercury dropped near the zero mark. I will use nearly any excuse to escape from a typewriter to the outdoors, so I told my wife I needed to do some field research, then went out and picked enough tender dock leaves to make a big dish of healthful greens for supper. Some of these young dock leaves were gathered near the head of a stream, fed by constant-temperature springs, from deep underground, which prevented their freezing and gave some protection to nearby vegetation. Others came from fields and roadsides where no such protection exists. Frost not only does not destroy this plant, it improves it. Young, newly grown dock leaves gathered when the nights are cold and frosty are mild and delicious. As the weather warms in the spring, I begin to notice that the dock greens we eat get less palatable. By the time we have had our last frost, they are so excruciatingly bitter as to be almost totally inedible, so gather your dock greens while the nights are still cold and the days nippy, if you want to enjoy them at their best.

While gathering the dock, I came on a spring-fed shallow pool covered with wild watercress, still doing nicely in the protection of these tempered waters. This time of the year, it reaches only an inch or so above the protecting spring water, making it rather tedious to pick, but in half an hour I had pinched off a quart of the tender, growing tips. Part of this will go into a tossed salad for tomorrow's dinner, and the remainder will be cooked with the dock tonight. Dock loses less bulk in cooking than most green leafy vegetables, and a small quantity will make a big dish of greens. Tonight we will cook the dock and the watercress together, in very little water, for about 15 minutes, then the greens will be drained, chopped, and seasoned with salt, butter, minced raw onion, some crumbled crisp bacon, and thin slices of hard-cooked egg. This will make a hearty supper dish that I would enjoy for taste alone, even if it weren't fairly bulging with all those healthful vitamins and minerals.

You don't have to follow my recipe slavishly in order to enjoy dock greens. The young, tender leaves, gathered while the weather is still cold, can be cooked in any way you would use spinach. Many cooks like to combine dock with other greens, wild or domestic. Watercress, dandelion, wild mustard, and winter-cress are favorites for these combinations and can usually be found while dock is still at its best. Many like to add a little cider vinegar or pepper sauce to dock greens as they are eaten. Some may object to the slight astringency in these greens and refuse to eat them unless they are creamed. The protein in milk combines with the tannin in dock leaves and removes the last trace of astringency. To make Creamed Dock, cook the greens, either alone or mixed in any proportions with other wild greens, then drain and chop. To cream 2 cups of these chopped greens, melt a tablespoon of butter in a saucepan, add a tablespoon of flour, and mix thoroughly. Add the greens and ½ cup of rich milk. Stir and cook until well mixed and slightly thickened. Add salt and pepper to taste, and you will have an appetizing dish ready to serve. A few people may find dock greens mildly laxative, but this is less likely to happen than with common rhubarb, to which dock is closely related.

The dark-brown seeds, which are really little dry fruits, are produced so abundantly on dock in late summer and fall that one wishes there was some good use for them besides adding them to dried-flower arrangements. Although this plant was originally introduced into America from Europe, it spread westward faster than did the white man, and there are reports that some tribes of western Indians formerly used these brown seeds to make an edible meal or flour. That would seem a logical use, since this plant is closely related to domestic buckwheat, from which the widely appreciated buckwheat flour is made.

To test this use I gathered about a peck of the winged seeds, just stripping them from the seedstalks with my hand. I rubbed them between my hands to remove the thin, diaphanous wings, a process that reduced my haul to less than half its original bulk. The seeds were winnowed by pouring them from one container to another in a breeze to clean them, then ground in a hand gristmill. The flour seemed very chaffy, so I sifted it, first through a fine flour sifter, then through a piece of even finer-meshed curtain material. This left me with about two cups of sifted flour, closely resembling buckwheat flour. I made some "buckwheat" cakes, using half this dock flour and half regular wheat flour. They were good enough, almost as good as those made of real buckwheat. My verdict: a good pancake flour if regular cereal grains are not available, but ordinarily not worth the trouble it takes to prepare it.

The medicinal part of curled dock is the long, yellow root, which still remains official in the *U.S. Dispensatory*. It is listed in the old herbals as a bitter tonic, astringent, gentle laxative and alterative. The bright-yellow color of the root betrays the presence of considerable vitamin A. Another active agent, rumicin, has been isolated and named. This root absolutely defies any effort to pull it up, so it must be dug from the ground. A long, slender spade is the best tool for this operation. The root should be thoroughly scrubbed, all side roots trimmed off, the main root split into two halves, and the pieces laid on paper, rounded side down, and dried in an airy room. I have tried three home remedies made of this root, an infusion, a syrup, and a salve.

The simple infusion, or dock-root tea, is made by pouring 1 pint of boiling water over ½ ounce of fine-shaved, dried dock root. Allow it to steep until cool, then strain, and discard the spent dock root. Keep the infusion in the refrigerator until used. A dose is a wine-glassful, unsweetened, a half-hour before breakfast every morning; it is supposed to be gently laxative, to tone up the system, purify the blood, and stimulate the appetite.

Dock syrup is a little stronger. A half-pound of the root is boiled in a pint of water until the liquid is reduced to 1 cupful. Strain and discard the spent root, and to the liquid add 1 cup of honey and stir until you have a homogeneous syrup. Taken a teaspoonful at a time, whenever needed, this is an excellent remedy for a cough, tickling throat, or mild irritation of the upper bronchial passages.

Cooked dock root has long had a reputation for curing an itch on man, and mange, saddle sores, and other external conditions on animals. The following recipe for dock salve, for external use, was adapted from an old English formula. Boil fresh dock root in vinegar just to cover until the root is soft and most of the vinegar has boiled away. Cool until it can be handled, then put the cooked dock root through a sieve or colander to remove the fiber. Combine 1 part dockroot pulp and 2 parts petroleum jelly, then work in enough dry, powdered sulfur to make the salve the proper consistency. This ointment seemed to quickly clear up a spot of itchy rash that developed on the back of my head, and also cured a mangy-looking spot between the ears of my cat. I fully realize these two instances do not comprise sufficiently comprehensive tests to prove anything, so if you make dock salve it will have to be on this meager evidence, the words of the ancient herbalists, and on your own faith in herbal remedies.

There are a number of other species of dock common in this country besides *Rumex crispus*. None of these is poisonous or harmful, and once you have become thoroughly familiar with one species you can easily recognize and sort out the others if you wish to pursue this subject. These different species really do not have to be distinguished, for the young leaves of all of them can be eaten, and the roots can all be used in making the home remedies described above. I have tried most species of dock that grow in the Middle Atlantic States, but I found none better than the common curled dock that is so abundant, and so neglected, throughout our land.

37. What I Do with the Blaspheme-vine and Indian Cucumber

O NE DAY in early summer I was leading a nature club on a walk, teaching them to identify wild-food plants. In the group was a man seventy-three years old, who said that he had been up until 3 A.M. the night before, teaching some young people Russian dancing. Despite the late hours and strenuous exercise of the night before, he was as fresh and chipper as anyone in the group, and could outwalk, outclimb, and outgather any of the young people who were along. Everyone wanted to know the secret of his perpetual youth, and he maintained, very seriously, that it was due to eating certain wild foods, fresh and green, when they were in season, and drinking herb wine and elderberry wine in the winter.

When pressed to point out the herbs that had such a magical effect, the elderly gentleman led us to a patch of tangled greenbrier, *Smilax rotundifolia*, and began gathering the tender young shoots of new growth that terminated the stout vines. These, with the tiny, unrolling new leaves and green tendrils still intact, were passed around for everyone to taste, and all agreed that they would make a salad well worth the eating, whether they were a fountain of youth or not. Our mentor said he ate a handful of these tasty shoots every day throughout the season that they were available. He credited much of his health and vigor to this vine, and said that he believed he could stay young and vigorous until he was a hundred years old if only he could

238

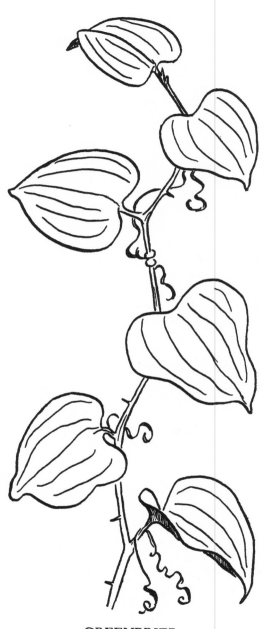

GREENBRIER

get greenbrier shoots the year round. When we stopped at noon to eat our box lunches, he pulled from his pack a bottle of his herb wine and another of his elderberry wine. We all sampled these, and agreed that this man, seventy-three years young, had discovered some exceedingly pleasant ways of keeping his youth.

GREENBRIER, CATBRIER, BULLBRIER, OR BLASPHEME-VINE
(Smilax, several species)

I had met the greenbrier before. As children we used to like the barely unrolling young leaves as pleasant, between-meal nibbles, calling them bread-and-butter for no reason that I can now imagine, for they certainly didn't taste like bread and butter. On being reintroduced to this plant by the youthful old man I started experimenting with it. The tender green shoots begin appearing about the first of May, are most plentiful in June, and can be found in gradually decreasing numbers until about the end of August. Be sure to pick only the tender, growing ends, taking them only as far down the vine as they will snap easily in two between the fingers. If, while gathering them, you become entangled in the old, woody vines with their fierce prickles, you will understand why the greenbriers are also called "blaspheme-vine."

The tender shoots are from three to six inches long and from a fourth to three-eighths of an inch in diameter, with several pairs of young, developing leaves and as many curling green tendrils. They really need no preparation whatever, and when on a picnic or hike I often gather a handful and eat them as a salad with my sandwiches. The texture is tender and crisp, while the flavor is slightly acid and very pleasant. At home I often gather some greenbrier shoots from the woodland across from my house, slice them fine crosswise, and add them to a tossed salad.

They can also be used as a cooked vegetable. Bound in serving-size bundles and boiled or steamed, as one does asparagus, they are excellent served hot with hollandaise sauce, or they can be boiled, then chilled and served with mayonnaise or French dressing. If greenbrier is a medicine, it is one of the most pleasant medicines to take that I know of, for I find it a very palatable food.

Several of the herbals list greenbrier as an alterative, an almost obsolete medical term that means, as nearly as I can figure out, a medicine that gradually makes the body healthier. Greenbrier is also a mild diuretic, and imparts to the urine a little of the same odor that is so noticeable after eating asparagus. So far as I know, this plant has never been explored to see what vitamins and minerals it contains, but from its bright yellow-green color and acid flavor, I would judge that it is fairly rich in vitamins A and C. Whether it is nutrients, or a drug, that gives greenbrier its healthful qualities, I cannot say, but whatever it is, it seems to be perfectly harmless, for I have eaten large quantities of this vegetable for long periods of time with no ill effects.

There are several species of greenbrier growing in this country, but all have a close family resemblance, and the green, tender shoots of all are edible. The old stems are slender, woody and green, freely branching and climbing by tendrils. Some stems may be more than thirty feet long, but little more than a quarter-inch in diameter. They usually climb over trees, brush or fences, but sometimes form dense, impenetrable thickets where they climb over one another. The old leaves are hard, tough, and leathery. The fruit is a blackish inedible berry, about a quarter-inch in diameter, borne in small umbels or clusters. It is only the very young shoots and the tips of the growing ends of the older vines that are crisp and tender, and these rapidly become woody and hard, so gather your greenbrier young, or not at all. Fortunately, these tender tips can be found over quite a long season in spring and summer. I find that I can recognize a cluster of greenbrier from a distance by their stems, which stay green summer and winter.

To distinguish the most common species of American greenbriers from one another, look at the leaves. *Smilax rotundifolia*, the most common greenbrier in the middle states, has heart-shaped pointed leaves about two inches across and three inches long. It is found from southern New England to Georgia, and west to Missouri and Texas. Over this same range one also finds S. *glauca*, a closely related species that can be identified by its fiddle-shaped leaves that are quite white, or whitish, underneath. S. *Bona-nox* also occurs over this same range, and it, too, has fiddle-shaped leaves, but they are green on both sides. S. *laurifolia* is called "bamboo vine" in some sections, and because it has the fiercest prickles of them all and grows in impenetrable thickets, it is the species most often called "blaspheme-vine." It has slender, oblong leaves, three to five inches long, that become very stiff and hard when fully mature. It is found in sandy pine barrens from southern New Jersey to Florida and west to Arkansas and Louisiana. And finally there is S. *tamnoides,* a southern species, found from Virginia to Florida, which is easily recognized because its stems are unarmed, or bear only a few very weak prickles. It is by far the most pleasant species to encounter. It is called "China root" in some sections, because of its large, tuberous roots, but you will hear all these species called "greenbrier," "catbrier," and "bullbrier" indiscriminately in most sections.

Both S. *tamnoides* and S. *Bona-nox* have another claim to fame besides their edible young shoots. These two species have fleshy, tuberous roots, and from these roots the southern Indian tribes prepared some of their favorite foodstuffs. Several early explorers reported this use of smilax, beginning with Captain John Smith, in his *Generall Historie of Virginia,* published in 1626. His directions for preparing it say to "cut it in small peeces, then stampe & straine it with water," and add that "boyled [it] makes a gelly good to eate." William Bartram, the great Quaker naturalist, in his *Travels Through North and South Carolina,* published in 1791, clarifies these directions a bit. He apparently actually observed the Indians at this task, and he says the roots were pounded, washed in water, and strained, and that the *powdery sediment* when dried formed a fine reddish flour. It was from this flour that the "gelly" of Captain Smith was made, and Bartram also says that the flour was used to make bread or cakes that were fried in bear's fat, and that the flour was used to thicken soups.

Many naturalists and writers of the 19th and 20th centuries have mentioned this use of these tuberous roots, but all of them seem to have drawn their information from Smith and Bartram. Apparently no one has tried to make this food in recent times, and when I had a yen to try this savage dish and set out to process some of the roots, I found out why; it's just too dam much work. The root is pounded, washed, and strained—and when you say it quickly, it sounds pretty easy, but wait until you try it! Remember, it is the sediment that settles in the bottom of the wash water that we want, so the pounding has to be thorough enough to loosen this edible part from the woody fibers that are strained out and thrown away. The Indians must have used large mortars and heavy pestles for this pounding; I finally had to take my roots to a farm shop and pound them on the anvil with a blacksmith's hammer. I washed the food from the fibers in a tub of cold water that I brought right into the shop, and when any root refused to give up its food, I gave it a second pounding.

Beating, loosening, and washing a few pounds of these tubers took a half-day's hard work. I strained out the fibers and allowed the washings to set for half an hour, then found that the edible parts had settled to the bottom and the wash water had become clear. I carefully decanted off the water, then spread the settlings on some trays and put them in the sun to dry. After several days, the water had evaporated and the settlings could be crumbled by hand into a fine meal. When the roots were first dug they were white inside and outside, but on exposure to air they began to turn a rusty-reddish color, and by the time the meal had dried, it was a bright rusty-red.

I found that 2 heaping tablespoons of this red meal, boiled for 10 minutes in 2 cups of water, would, on cooling, harden into a jelly-like Greenbrier Pudding that was pretty good when eaten with honey and cream. The flavor was bland and somewhat flat, but I found it improved when flavored by boiling a bit of sassafras root with it. I wonder whether I was the first to make this "gelly" since the 18th century?

Next I made a stew of marrowy beef shinbone, seasoned it with a handful of garlicky wild leeks and thickened it with a half-cup of the red smilax meal. This was excellent, with a wild, unusual but very good flavor. When I tried making meal cakes of this red meal alone they were dry and poor in taste and texture, but when I mixed the meal half-and-half with wheat flour, they improved considerably. The recipe I finally worked out for Smilax Cakes calls for 1 cup red meal, 1 cup flour, 1 teaspoon soda, 1 slightly beaten egg, 3 tablespoons cooking oil, and 1 pint of buttermilk. This is mixed into a thin batter that is dropped by the spoonful on a not-too-hot griddle and lightly browned on both sides. We found these cakes so good with maple syrup or wild-fruit jams that the rest of our red smilax meal went this way.

When I turned to S. rotundifolia, it was a different story. This species came highly recommended, but failed to live up to its reputation. I have seldom told of my failures in this book, not because I didn't have them, nor because I want to conceal them, but because I am sure you are much more interested in what you can do with wild plants than in what you can't do. However, my attempt to use the roots of S. rotundifolia so plainly illustrates why I thought it necessary to repeat every experiment I read about, and personally to try every recipe I uncovered, that I decided to include it. In two books that I had formerly considered dependable I found directions for making jelly of these greenbrier roots. They correctly described the roots as long, cordlike and white, and mentioned that they would begin to turn a reddish color when exposed to the air, a phenomenon that I also observed. They explained that it was not absolutely necessary to powder these roots to make jelly of them, and claimed that they had made excellent jelly by merely cutting these roots in fine pieces, boiling them for an hour, then straining and adding sugar to the liquid, and boiling again for a few minutes. They even described the color, texture, and flavor of the resulting jelly.

These directions were so explicit and clear that I had no doubt that S. *rotundifolia* would perform as advertised, so I decided to make some of this jelly as a demonstration to a class of boys I was instructing on the use of wild food. We were a bit surprised to find that these "roots" were really hard, woody rhizomes, or underground stems, and that the real roots were fine, tough and wiry, extending downward from the numerous joints on these rhizomes. "Not absolutely necessary to powder these roots . . ." indeed! Powdering these flexible, woody rhizomes would be like trying to powder a walking cane; possible for a determined person with adequate equipment and unlimited time, but most of us wouldn't tackle such a job. These writers claimed that they "merely cut the rootstocks in fine pieces . . ." but let me warn you there is nothing "mere" about cutting these so-called "rootstocks" in fine pieces.

A dozen of us with sharp knives finally reduced enough of these rootstocks to fine shavings to fill a small kettle. These shavings were duly covered with cold water and then put on to boil for the directed hour. The water did turn dark-colored, resembling strong tea. We strained the shavings from this water, added sugar in directed amounts, and put it back on to boil again. Nothing happened. The stuff refused to jell, no matter how much or how little sugar we added, how long we boiled it, or how long we cooled it. The flavor of the syrup we made this way wasn't bad, but it really wasn't anything to brag about, and it wouldn't jell under any circumstances that we could discover.

Recently, I wondered if the ground in which the catbriers grew could have had anything to do with this failure—or was it perhaps because we gathered the rhizomes in spring, rather than in the fall? I gathered a new supply of roots in late autumn, about two hundred miles from where I had collected the first ones. They yielded exactly the same results.

F. P. Porcher, in his book *Resources of the Southern Fields and Forests*, writes that Confederate soldiers used the roots of smilax to make a sort of root beer, which they called sarsaparilla, this name being either an amazing coincidence, or betraying the fact that some soldier had a more-than-ordinary knowledge of botany, for the real sarsaparilla is a tropical species of smilax. Porcher gave a recipe of sorts for this beverage, specifying the ingredients without giving quantities, and since I couldn't make jelly of *S. rotundifolia*, I decided to try to make beer.

I gathered about 3 pounds of the rhizomes and reduced them to shavings, added a cupful of ground, parched corn and ½ cup of sassafras-root bark, covered them with 1 gallon of cold water, then put it all on to boil for 1 hour. This liquid was strained to remove the solid parts, and, when it was lukewarm, I added a cup of molasses and a teaspoon of dry active yeast that I had dissolved in a little of the liquid. By evening it was beginning to bubble, so I bottled it in green ginger ale bottles and capped it with crown caps. After storing these in my dark cellar for a month, I chilled a bottle and opened it. It foamed like commercial root beer, and the flavor wasn't at all bad, in fact it was almost as good as the root beer I can buy at any store or hot dog stand for ten cents per bottle.

Next year I intend to eat a great many of the tender shoots of catbriers, partly because I like them, and partly to preserve any youth and health to which I can still lay claim. But in order to conserve my waning energy and save my easily lost temper I am going to leave the roots undug.

INDIAN CUCUMBER
(*Medeola virginiana*)

I hesitated a long time before mentioning this delightful wild food, for in order to enjoy it, a very decorative wild plant of the lily family must be destroyed. However, I have found that foragers and neo-primitive food gatherers are among the best conservationists, so I have decided our clan can be trusted with this information with no danger of extinction to the Indian cucumber. The conscientious nature-lover will dig this tasty, crisp root only from areas where the attractive plant is growing too thickly for its own good or when there is emergency need for the food it can provide.

The Indian cucumber grows in rich woods from Maine to Georgia and west to Minnesota. The aboveground part of the plant is a single slender stem, usually about a foot high, and about two-thirds of the way up its length it bears a circle of five to seven elongate leaves like the ribs of an umbrella, and at its summit another whorl of three (rarely four or five) much shorter leaves. Above these upper leaves appear the straw-colored flowers, each having three slender, recurved petals and six stamens. The flowers are followed by dark-purple berries, three-celled, with few seeds. The leaves become deeply suffused with purple in the late summer and fall. The plant springs from a horizontal, tuber-like root the size of a little finger. These roots are snow-white, crisp, tender, and delicious, with a distinct flavor of cucumber.

Despite its common name, I can find only one reference to its use by American Indians. Most writers on primitive Indian foods fail to mention it, which seems strange in view of its attractiveness, food value, and palatability. Here is one wild forest delicacy we can enjoy that was apparently overlooked by most of the Amerindian tribes, probably because they did not have cucumbers and therefore their tastes were not trained in this direction. I have tried it cooked and it is a pretty good vegetable when boiled and seasoned with butter and salt, but I prefer it raw as a woodland nibble or carried home and sliced into a tossed salad dressed with oil and vinegar.

The pronounced cucumber flavor of these crisp, white roots naturally led me to wonder how they would taste pickled. My rather lazy experiment along these lines worked perfectly. I simply mixed ½ cup of vinegar, ½ cup of water, a tablespoonful of salt, and a teaspoonful of sugar together cold. I put a flower-head of fresh dill in the bottom of a pint jar, dropped in a little red pepper and a clove of garlic, and packed the jar with well-washed roots, poured the liquid over them, and sealed the jar with a two-piece metal lid. About two months later, I opened the jar and found some of the nicest and crispest Wild Dill Pickles I ever tasted.

According to *Gray's Manual of Botany*, *Medeola virginiana* received its genus name from the Greek sorceress Medea, for its supposed medicinal virtues, but after searching through more than a

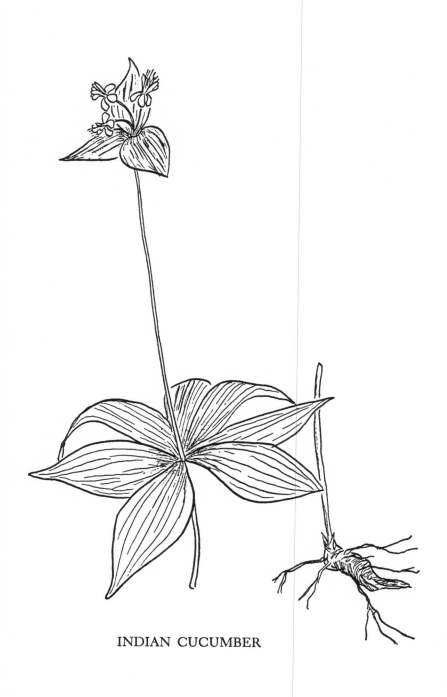

INDIAN CUCUMBER

dozen books on American medicinal herbs I cannot find mention of any medicinal use for it. Still I feel justified in discussing this interesting plant in a book on healthful herbs, for the mere sight of it will cure the beauty-starved eye of one who has been too long out of touch with nature. The crisp rootstock will cure the hunger of a man lost in the woods or a hiker who has strayed too far from his dining room, and when this root is sliced and properly dressed it will cure the banality with which altogether too many tossed salads are afflicted.

38. Jack-in-the-pulpit or Indian-turnip

(*Arisaema triphyllum*)

THIS interesting plant is also called "wakerobin," but I dislike this name as it tends to confuse it with the trilliums, several of which are also called "wakerobins." The two plants are unrelated. People more often ask me about the edible qualities of Jack-in-the-pulpit than about almost any other plant. This is probably because one of its most common folk names is Indian-turnip, and because this plant is so easily recognized that it is known to more people than almost any other wildflower. Even the "turnip" is known to many through hard experience, for a favorite trick of country boys is to offer a slice of the root, which looks eminently edible, to an unsuspecting victim. At first this root tastes sweet and palatable, then almost instantly starts to prickle and burn and soon sets the mouth and throat on fire.

The "Jack" is a perennial, springing anew each year from its starchy bulb or corm. It grows one to three feet high, bearing two long-stalked leaves, each composed of three ovate, pointed leaflets. These overshadow the conspicuous green- and purple-striped spathe, or hood, that rises on a separate stalk between them. The spathe curves in a broad canopy-like portion over the top of the club-shaped, upright spike, or spadix, two to three inches long, near the base of which, concealed by the encircling hood, are the minute flowers. This spike, standing in the canopied hood, so resembles a little priest standing in an enclosed pulpit, that it has given the plant its most common folk name, Jack-in-the-pulpit, but I wonder if the little preacher isn't warning of the hellfire contained in the turnip-like corm just below him. The flower is followed by an egg-shaped cluster of bright-red berries that ripen in late summer and are as fiery-hot as the corm.

Jack-in-the-pulpit grows in rich, low woods and damp places from Nova Scotia to Florida and west to Minnesota and Kansas. Most people have heard that the Indians used the turnip-shaped root of this plant for food, but very few realize the extent of the processing necessary to render it palatable. I recently read a book on how to enjoy living in the country, and it included a number of recipes for preparing wild plants. The author wrote of the acridity and pungency of the Indian-turnip, but then went on to say that these properties were completely dispelled by cooking, and that he and his family had often enjoyed boiled Indian turnips, finding them delicious. This statement caused me to lose all confidence in anything else the man had written. Surely he should have experimented at least once with cooking the corms of Jack-in-the-pulpit before making that statement, but obviously he didn't, or he has a tougher palate than mine. Had he merely written, "It is often *said* that cooking removes the acridity and pungency from Indian turnip," I would agree with him. It *is* often said, and often written, but usually by those who haven't tried it. I have boiled Indian turnips for hours, and they were still far too pungent for anyone to take even one bite of them. To eat a whole serving of such concentrated fire would not only be sheer torture, but would undoubtedly cause serious gastric disturbances.

Jack-in-the-pulpit belongs to the arum family, and all members of this family have acrid and peppery qualities that are caused by millions of microscopic raphides, or needle-like crystals of oxalate of lime, that crowd the fresh tissue. Many arums have large, fleshy roots that are rich in starch, and these are good-flavored if the prickling and burning propensities can be removed. Primitive tribes in many remote parts of the world have apparently independently discovered means of rendering these irritating crystals harmless, and have come to rely on members of the arum family as abundant sources of excellent food. These crystals are affected little, if at all, by boiling. However, dry heat, or prolonged drying, does cause the crystals to break down, and then the Indian-turnip is sweet and palatable. When I say prolonged drying, I mean prolonged. I cut some of the turnips in thin slices, like potato chips, and dried them in my attic. In three weeks they were perfectly dry, but still retained their fire when tasted. After two months, most of them were edible, but even then one would occasionally find one that would prickle the throat. After about five months, the peppery quality was completely dispelled, and the dried chips had an excellent flavor.

These long-dried Indian-Turnip Chips are very good with no further preparation than a short toasting to make them crisp. They can be eaten like potato chips, with or without flavorsome dips. Crumbled fine and boiled about 10 minutes, they make an excellent Jack-in-the-pulpit Cereal to be eaten with sugar and cream. Ground fine, they make a flour that can add a unique and delicious flavor, slightly reminiscent of cocoa, to cakes, cookies, muffins, rolls, and pancakes. The crumbled chips are easily ground in a coffee mill or hand grist-mill, or with a mortar and pestle. This flour, or meal, contains little or no gluten, and should be mixed, half and half, with regular wheat flour to give the products a pleasing texture.

As an example of its use, the following Jack-in-the-pulpit Cookies are favorites at our house. Cream 1 cup butter and ⅓ cup sugar. Add 1 teaspoon vanilla and 1 tablespoon water. Sift together 1 cup flour and 1 cup Jack-in-the-pulpit flour. Add this, with 1 cup chopped hickory-nut meats to other ingredients, and mix well. Shape into small balls the size of marbles and bake on ungreased cookie sheet for 20 minutes in a 325° oven. Pass them around warm or cold, and make no apologies. You can substitute black walnuts or wild pecans for the hickory nuts called for in this recipe and get some delightful variations in flavor. If you are not a purist, you can even use nuts from the store.

Medicinally, Jack-in-the-pulpit is described as a counterirritant, rubefacient, carminative, diaphoretic, and expectorant. I found the breakfast gruel described above listed as a good medicine for coughs and pulmonary consumption. I find it a palatable and nourishing food for healthy people, too, and prefer not to think of it as a medicine. If eating a bowl of it for breakfast also increases perspiration, loosens phlegm, and dispels gas, and if these things are good for me, so much the better, but the reason I eat Jack-in-the-pulpit Cereal is that I like it. In most cases, people who are sick would be benefited by getting some palatable but bland and easily digested food inside them, and that is exactly what this cereal is, aside from any drug benefits that might be there as pure bonus.

JACK-IN-THE-PULPIT

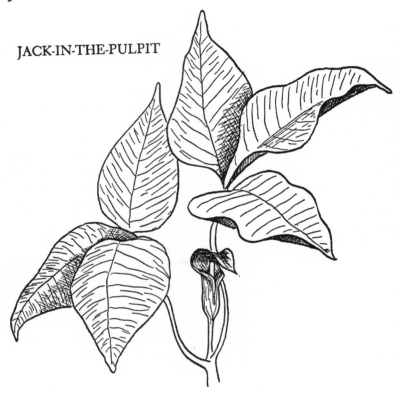

I find two medicinal uses listed for Jack-in-the-pulpit root that I am sure will never become popular with us. Some American Indians, when they had a headache, would apply the ground, freshly dried root to the forehead. This would cause sweating, and the sweating would cause the powder to sting and burn until the pain on the outside became so excruciating that one forgot the pain inside. This is the theory of the counterirritant, a technique that still finds some use in modern medicine, but nowadays we usually try to relieve a pain rather than merely trading it in on a new one.

The second use that sounds very painful to me is using a rolled paper to blow a small pinch of freshly dried and powdered Indian-turnip into the throats of children suffering from sore throat. The theory here is that the irritation of the powder acts as a rubefacient, drawing a copious flow of blood, with its healing and restoring powers, to the affected area. It might even have some healing effect, but the prickling and burning of the throat, especially a sensitive sore throat, must be torture. Probably the reason this was specified as a remedy for children is that the recipient of such a dose had to be small enough to be overpowered and forced to take it. I know it would take a very large and strong man to get me to submit to having fresh Jack-in-the-pulpit powder blown into my throat.

Because of the long drying necessary to make it edible, Indian-turnip is not useful as an emergency or survival food, nor can it be prepared as a camp dish during a short vacation. I am glad this handsome wildflower is not as tasty in the fresh state as it is after long preparation, otherwise the last Jack-in-the-pulpit root would long ago have disappeared down some gluttonous gullet. Only those patient and wise enough to remove its pungency are allowed to enjoy Jack-in-the-pulpit as food. The plant should not be gathered indiscriminately, but this does not mean that avid wild-food enthusiasts cannot select a few choice turnips from a thick stand to prepare some dip-chips for future "wild parties" or to grind some flour to make "wild" cookies to serve with some of the wild teas described elsewhere in this book. Conservation doesn't mean non-use, and it is the users of this plant who will come to its rescue when the species is threatened. The chief danger to little Jack is not from those few nature-lovers who want to use an occasional corm for food, but from the horde of "improvers," who, in the name of reclamation, want to level all the hills and fill in all the swamps. It is the ones who know, love, and occasionally use the Indian-turnip who will try to see to it that suitable habitats remain where this jolly little priest in his tiny pulpit can continue to preach about the eternal miracle of nature's resurrection every spring.

39. The Odorous Skunk-cabbage

(*Symplocarpus foetidus*)

THE SKUNK-CABBAGE is the best spring harbinger of them all, and along the stream that is across the road from my home, it is the very first spring plant to appear, pushing through the wet muck almost as soon as the ground has thawed. The first part to appear is the fleshy, leathery, shell-shaped spathe, as large as—and shaped much as—your two cupped hands. It is striped and mottled in fascinating patterns of dark and light green, deep purple, and dark red. Inside the spathe is a globular mass of insignificant and not very pretty lavender-colored flowers, their color often obscured by the many straw-colored anthers bearing heavy loads of yellow pollen.

A week or two after the first flowers are seen, the leaves make their appearance, pushing through the mold in tightly rolled cones, yellowish-green in color. When one of these tight cones of leaves is cut or broken, one will immediately see why it is called a cabbage, for it closely resembles a cut head of ordinary cabbage, while the odor that will greet you leaves no doubt whatever why this name is preceded by the adjective *skunk*. Frankly, this plant stinks. The bruised or cut leaves smell like a skunk, the cut stem smells like a mixture of mustard and rotten, raw onions, and the flowers smell like carrion. The newborn leaves soon unroll and continue to expand and grow in a completely uninhibited manner, becoming from one to two feet high and about as broad by the first of June. They are called "elephant-ears" in some sections because of their large size.

Of course, the skunk-cabbage is totally unrelated to the true cabbage. It is an arum, closely akin to the Jack-in-the-pulpit. It has an extensive range, being found in swamps and marshy places from eastern Quebec to western Ontario and south to Missouri and Georgia.

Probably because of its wide availability and great abundance, and its succulent, edible appearance, skunk-cabbage seems to have captured the imaginations of nearly all writers on wild foods and herbal medicines, but when I read some of the things these writers have said I sometimes wonder if they are talking about the same plant I know. I was able to find five different accounts of the use of skunk-cabbage as food, all highly recommending it as a vegetable, with some of them almost going into ecstasies about its palatability. All recommended exactly the same method of preparation, using the tightly rolled cones of young leaves, cutting and cooking them like cabbage, except that they were boiled in two or more waters with a pinch of soda added to the first water. They all recommended seasoning it like other vegetables, with butter, salt, and pepper.

While these accounts showed more than a little evidence of having been copied from one another, or from a common source, all the authors claimed to have had firsthand experience with preparing and eating this food. All agreed that during the cooking no trace of the disagreeable odor was given off, and they were unanimous in pronouncing it good.

With that kind of recommendation from reputable authors I would willingly try any experiment. I gathered some of the tightly folded cones of leaves and set out to cook this palatable dish. The first thing that went wrong was that smell, but maybe they were right when they said, "No trace of odor was given off," for that odor certainly couldn't be described as a "trace." It was thick, heavy, and foul, and continued to be given off throughout the cooking, through first, second, and third waters, each with its recommended pinch of soda. By the time I was finished cooking, the kitchen smelled as if it had been visited by an angry skunk. I aired out the place, sprayed kitchen deodorant, seasoned the vegetable, and boldly sampled it. It tasted exactly like it smelled, and I certainly wouldn't describe that taste as pleasing. After chewing and swallowing one bite, I started to take another, but about then my mouth and throat began to burn as though I had taken a bite of raw Jack-in-the-pulpit. The burning wasn't really torturous, but it was uncomfortable. I persuaded six other people to sample this dish, telling them only what the others had said about its palatability, but they were unanimous in rejecting a second bite. I lost the friendship of one little girl who before had always been a willing taster of the wild-food concoctions I was constantly cooking. She not only disliked boiled skunk-cabbage, but considered my persuading her to take a bite of it a vicious and unforgivable practical joke.

I don't give up easily on a wild food that comes so highly recommended. One of the references indicated that the plants were apt to vary, some being quite mild and sweet, and others being smelly and peppery. I wondered if I had merely been unlucky in the plants I had selected, so I drove to a swamp several miles away and gathered a new supply, but these gave exactly the same results when cooked. About this time I had occasion to go on a trip to a country place about two hundred miles away. While there I gathered some more young skunk-cabbage leaves for a third experiment. Same smell, same taste, same burning sensation, same total inedibility. I'd had it. Maybe those other authors know where the good skunk-cabbage grows, but I don't.

The same books say that the Indians made a palatable and nutritious breadstuff of the roots of skunk-cabbage, so I turned my attention to this part of the plant, with somewhat better success. The roots are about two inches thick and about one foot long, and they are firmly anchored by numerous cordlike side rootlets. The easiest way to dig them is to run a sharp spade down all sides of the primary root to cut its anchor cords, then dig off the top layer of muck and grasp the root and pull it out. If you try pulling on the plant, it will only break off at the top of the root, which is usually about six inches below the surface. Take the roots to a stream or pond to wash away the clinging mud. On cutting into these roots, I found they were composed of a fairly well-defined rind or peel, to which the white rootlets were attached, and a white, starchy core. I peeled the roots and cut the starchy cores in thin slices and put them to dry on clean papers in my large, hot, airy attic. At the same time I decided to see if the cabbage could be improved by drying, so cut a number of the cones of tightly rolled leaves in thin slices and put them to dry on separate papers. While working with these products I was acutely aware of the skunky odor, which seems to permeate every part of the plant. After a few weeks of drying, the odor disappeared, and, as with other arums, it seems to be the drying and aging that dispels the biting pungency and acridity that makes them inedible in the fresh state.

After one month of drying, I ground some of the crisp root-chips in my hand gristmill for a trial. Mixed half-and-half with wheat flour they made a Skunk-Cabbage Pancake that tasted good enough, but within a minute of eating it I felt the now familiar burning and prickling in my throat. I put the rest of the root-chips in a muslin bag and hung them from an attic rafter for further aging. That autumn, six months after they were lifted from the ground, I tried again. I ground them fine, mixed the meal half-and-half with wheat flour and again made pancakes. This time I experienced no burning sensation whatever, and the pancakes were something special. The flavor was pronounced, but very pleasant, a bit like cocoa but different. With butter and maple syrup these pancakes were unusually good. I had finally discovered a way to make a palatable skunk-cabbage product.

Encouraged by this success, I decided to try the sliced cabbage that had been drying since spring. This was dry and crisp and easily crumbled when handled. I decided to try making an old-fashioned Herb-Meat Cabbage Pudding of it. As there were only my wife and I to eat it, I made it small, 1 cup crumbled, dried skunk-cabbage, 2 slices whole-wheat bread, 1 medium-sized onion, minced, ¼ cup raw rice, ½ cup pork sausage, a can of undiluted mushroom soup, and half a teaspoon caraway seed. This was all mixed thoroughly, tied in a cloth, and boiled for about 90 minutes. It came out round as a cannonball, and when served with a sauce made of a half-cup of soy sauce and a teaspoon of hot Chinese mustard, stirred together, it was eminently edible, in fact, delicious. I'm sure a clever cook could find other ways of using dehydrated skunk-cabbage, and next year I'm going to dry more.

Skunk-cabbage is found in nearly every list of medicinal herbs I examined, and all seem to agree on its uses. This could mean that it is a widely accepted remedy with well-attested efficacy in certain illnesses, or it could merely mean that we herbalists tend to copy from one another. Skunk-cabbage once won a place in the official *U.S. Pharmacopoeia* and is still listed in the *U.S. Dispensatory*. Reputed properties are listed as emetic, stimulant, antispasmodic, and narcotic, and there is usually appended a warning that overdoses are likely to cause nausea, vomiting, dizziness, and dimness of sight. This seems to indicate that there is some powerful drug in the fresh plant that is dispelled on drying, for the dried products had no unpleasant side effects whatever. The part used in herbal medicine is the freshly dried root, 1 ounce of the root being covered with boiling water, steeped for ½ hour, then strained, and sweetened with 2 tablespoons honey. This tea is given cold, 1 ounce at a time, three times a day for cough, catarrh, asthma, or bronchitis. I tried this medicine, and three doses in one day seemed to cause no ill effects; on one occasion, it did seem to relieve a night cough that had probably been brought on by too much smoking.

The skunky smell of this infusion would repel most people, and the taste is pretty gruesome, even with the added honey. It is said that the Indians used skunk-cabbage to cover up even worse tastes and smells in their medicines, which leads me to wonder just how bad their medicines tasted and smelled. They also used the powdered freshly dried root as a styptic to stop bleeding from minor cuts and scratches, a logical use, since its astringency would have this effect. Summed up, skunk-cabbage seems to furnish a useful medicine for some complaints and is a very passable food plant for those willing to complete the lengthy processing necessary to make it edible.

If you still insist on experimenting with skunk-cabbage, be sure you have correctly identified it, for there is another large-leaved green plant found growing in low places, often intermingled with skunk-cabbage, that is very poisonous. This is green hellebore, *Veratrum viride*, also called Indian poke, and by some, mistakenly, called skunk-cabbage, making it very dangerous to depend on local information when you are trying to distinguish between these two plants.

There is really little excuse for confusing these quite dissimilar plants. Both grow in low places and both have very large green leaves, but there the resemblance ends. The leaves of skunk-cabbage grow directly from the top of the root, that is, the plant is stalkless, while the leaves of green hellebore grow from a central stalk. Skunk-cabbage leaves are smooth and moist to the touch, and green hellebore leaves are longitudinally fluted, or pleated. Green hellebore completely lacks the characteristic odor with which skunk-cabbage offends our noses.

With these major differences it would seem unlikely that anyone could confuse these two plants, and yet, I have known of two cases where people ate green hellebore thinking it was skunk-cabbage. In one case a man gathered and cooked a little of what his neighbors called "skunk-cabbage" as an experiment. Since it proved to be very unpalatable, he and his wife took only one bite apiece, but this was enough to make both very ill, and they spent several hours vomiting, retching, and gagging, but both recovered. In the other case, a man with much enthusiasm for wild food, but little experience in using it, decided to prepare a wild meal for his friends. Misled by those writers who insist that cooked fresh skunk-cabbage makes a palatable dish, he gathered a quantity of what he thought was skunk-cabbage and cooked it to serve as a vegetable at his "wild party." His "vegetable" would have been inedible, to my taste, even if he had prepared the right plant, but he picked green hellebore by mistake. The wild dinner progressed no further than the vegetable course, for everyone became ill, and even with the help of a hastily summoned doctor, they had a pretty uncomfortable time of it. They all recovered, but none of them have shown much enthusiasm for wild food since then.

Obviously, green hellebore is not for eating, but it is a drug plant of no mean order, appearing in both the U.S. *Pharmacopoeia* and the *National Formulary*. Though valuable in the hands of a competent physician, green hellebore is far too drastic and dangerous a drug for the amateur herbalist to use in experiments; it is strictly not for use in home remedies. The parts used medicinally are the roots and rhizomes, and these yield several alkaloids, the most important of which is *protoveratrine*, which in extremely small doses can dramatically lower blood pressure, reduce the pulse rate, induce sweating, and lower the body temperature. It is easy to see how an overdose of such powerful medicine could cause death. Fortunately, the herb is also an emetic in overdoses, so it is usually spontaneously vomited, and actual death from green hellebore is rare, but it takes very little to induce a very uncomfortable sickness.

It was those master herbalists, the American Indians, who first discovered the powers of green hellebore and introduced this active drug to modern medicine. There is no doubt that this medicine was misused. A doctor finding a hard, rapid pulse and a high fever would administer a dose of *Elixir of Veratrum viride*, and quickly bring these symptoms within normal range. However, what was obtained was only a simulation of normality, for green hellebore did not correct the conditions that caused the symptoms, but merely exerted a powerful drug action on the centers controlling the symptoms. It was later realized that such symptoms were often indications that the body was working extra hard to correct its own malfunctioning, and a drug that interfered with the processes which were causing these symptoms only delayed diagnosis and recovery. This new attitude caused green hellebore to fall into disuse for a time. A textbook of pharmacology published in 1941 says of *Veratrum viride*: "The drug is practically obsolete today and enjoys a deserved oblivion."

But green hellebore wasn't that easily assigned to oblivion. What this doctor thought was a permanent passing turned out to be a very temporary eclipse. In 1952, a doctor began research on another herb that came directly from folk medicine. This was the now famous *rauwolfia*, or Indian snakeroot, which had been used in the herbal medicine of India for thousands of years. This doctor found that snakeroot would lower blood pressure, but it was a slow-acting drug. It occurred to him that he had another blood-pressure-reducing drug close at hand, so he added small amounts of green hellebore to the medicine and found the results were good. Since high blood pressure is one of the more serious factors in diseases of the heart and circulatory system, which are, by far, the leading causes of death in this country, this was a tremendously important discovery. Note that here a new "miracle drug" was produced by wedding the herbal folklore of the East Indians with that of the American Indians. Let modern medicine acknowledge the debt that it owes to those ancient medicine men who first discovered the powers that reside in these ordinary-appearing wild herbs.

40. Chufa or Nut-grass

(*Cyperus esculentus*)

THE CHUFA is a fine food and medicinal herb with an almost universal distribution, being found in Europe, Africa, Asia, and America. In North America it is found from New Brunswick to Minnesota and southward to Florida and Texas, and on the Pacific Coast, it grows wild from Alaska to Mexico. The botanical name means "edible sedge," and the chufa is related to the tules and bulrushes. It has grasslike leaves at the base, and its stout, triangular seedstalk rises one to two feet. Near its top is another circle of leaves, similar to the base leaves in shape, but smaller, and above these stem leaves is the flower cluster, consisting of five to eight rays, each bearing numerous little flat spikelets. The edible part is borne underground, and while it is called a nut, it is really a small tuber, about half an inch long, dark-colored and wrinkled.

The chufa likes rich, wet, alluvial soil, but if this soil happens to be heavy, sticky, and hard to dig, the chufa compounds the difficulty by bearing only a few tiny tubers and scattering these widely by producing them on long stolons so that they hide some distance from the parent plant. Chufa plants can be plentiful in such places, and yet a man could starve to death trying to live on the tubers he could collect, even if he spent all his time digging for them. On the other hand, where the soil is light, sandy, and easy to dig, the chufa is likely to bear huge crops of larger tubers only an inch or so below the surface and concentrated right under and around the plant. In such places, one can sometimes merely grasp all the grasslike leaves and stout stems and pull up the plant, bringing up at least three-fourths of the nuts with it, without digging at all. Never mind about destroying a decorative and useful plant. Every one of those little tubers that are inevitably left in the ground, no matter how closely you harvest, is perfectly capable of producing an entire new plant that will ripen another crop of nuts in a year. Pick the little tubers from their stolons, wash them to remove any clinging dirt, spread them on clean papers, and as soon as they are dry they are ready to be eaten.

Chufa eating has a venerable history. The ancient Egyptians enjoyed chewing on chufas and developed cultivated strains of this wild plant about five thousand years ago. All classes must have relished them, for the Pharaohs wouldn't be caught dead without a supply of chufas. When their tombs are opened, the archeologists usually find a quantity of mummified chufas within easy reach of the preserved corpses. Apparently they distrusted the quality of the food they could expect in the afterlife and wanted to take along something they liked.

Chufas are still prized in some parts of Spain, North Africa, Ethiopia, and a few other parts of the world. About a hundred years ago there was a flurry of excitement over chufas in this country, when it was thought they might prove a profitable crop in our own sandy Southland. Cultivated varieties were introduced from Africa, and they produced tremendous crops, but the labor of harvesting them was too great, and since our people hadn't been educated to appreciate chufas, the demand for them was too small. However, the planters soon discovered that it was easier to start raising chufas than to quit. The African strains were of the same species as our native chufas, and both found the South a pleasant place to grow. They are so persistent and so prolific that the chufa is today, in many areas, despised as a weed. There is no integration problem among plants, so today, when you harvest wild chufas in the South, you neither know nor care whether they had African or American ancestors, or both.

I believe the time has come to make another attempt at raising chufas commercially on a large scale. The best cultivated strains in suitable soil will produce up to two hundred bushels of these tiny tubers per acre. Peanut-harvesting machinery could be adapted to chufas, or new machinery could be designed and built. It is easier to introduce a new food in America today than it has ever been before. Chufas would merely have to be rolled, shredded, puffed, or toasted, then packaged in cellophane-wrapped boxes and sold as just one more of those cereals of unidentifiable origin that appear on American breakfast tables. Or, the little tubers could be dried, ground into flour,

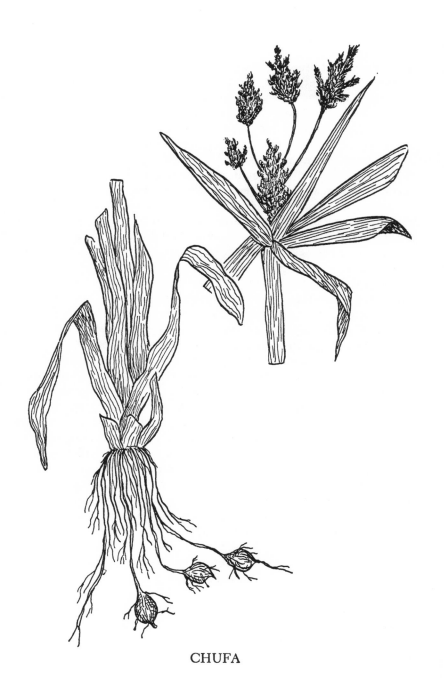

CHUFA

and blended with some of the package mixes with which the modern housewife does her baking. Maybe chufas would give some of these products a little taste.

To one who has never eaten chufas the first one is always a surprise. It isn't crunchy, like a nut, but crinkles between the teeth, and as it is chewed it yields copious amounts of sweet white milk. The flavor? Well, flavors are notoriously hard to describe, but let's say it is in between the flavors of coconut and almond, with a tang or two all its own. Very few dislike it, even at the first taste.

Medicinally, chufa is considered merely a good digestive and nutritive, containing no dangerous drugs whatever, so that it can be taken freely by the sick and the well, children and adults. The Spaniards make a beverage called *horchata de chufas*, which they consider an agreeable and health-giving refreshment for invalids and convalescents, as well as being appreciated by those who have nothing whatever wrong with them. The Spanish recipe involves too much work as it stands, but a modern electric blender can marvelously lighten this labor. Soak ½ pound of washed tubers in cold water for about 2 days, then drain. Put 1 quart of water and ¼ cup of sugar in your blender, then, running it at high speed, feed in the chufas. Blend until the tubers are cut so fine that the liquid is practically homogenized. Strain through a clean cloth, and it is ready to drink. This is a white, milky liquid, sweet and smooth, with an excellent flavor. I made another batch, using ½ cup of sugar, and froze it to a smooth consistency in an ice cream freezer; it made a tasty Chufa Sherbet.

If chufa tubers are roasted until they are a very dark brown all through, then pulverized in a blender or coffee mill, they make a very palatable hot drink when brewed exactly as you do coffee. This brew tastes more like some of the roasted cereal health-food drinks than it does like coffee, but it is a good hot beverage of that class. I have several times tried Chufa Coffee for dinner when I was afraid that real coffee would keep me awake too long, and have always found it a pleasant drink. It contains no harmful stimulants and can be freely given to children who insist on having "coffee" when the adults do.

Candied Chufas are a tasty nibble, probably more wholesome than most commercial candies, and easy to make. Soak the tubers for 2 days in cold water, then drain. Put equal parts by measure of soaked chufas, sugar, and water in a saucepan, and simmer until the chufas

are tender and clear-looking. Drain off the syrup and let the chufas
dry for a day, then roll them in granulated sugar and store in the
refrigerator until they are eaten, which won't be long.

All writers who mention this plant give high praise to the quality
of the flour that can be ground from the dried tubers, and my own
experiments did not contradict them. Fresh chufas cannot be ground
until they are thoroughly dried, and this is best done in a slow oven
with the door propped slightly open so moisture can escape. The idea
is to dry the chufas until they are friable without cooking them too
much. It will take several hours, the exact time depending on how
dry the chufas were when put into the oven. When a cooled tuber
will break apart when hit a light blow with a hammer, instead of
merely being mashed, they are ready to grind. These toasted chufas
can be ground in a hand grist mill or a coffee grinder with the burrs
set as closely as possible together, or a small quantity can be ground
in a food chopper with a fine plate, or even in that electric blender
that seems so necessary to a neo-primitive food gatherer.

Chufa is one of the finest-tasting and most nourishing wild bread-
stuffs I ever tried. Mixed half-and-half with wheat flour it is very
good in biscuits, muffins, griddle cakes, and cookies, and mixed with
cornmeal it makes an excellent Indian Pudding. Another possible
commercial outlet for chufas would be as a truly palatable health-
food flour, for according to one recent source this flour contains vitamin C and a very active fat-splitting enzyme of the lipase family.

One of the best things I made of chufa flour was a batch of almost
candy-like Chufa Cookies. Cream 1 cup softened butter with ⅓ cup
of sugar and add about 4 teaspoons of water. Add 1 cup of wheat
flour and 1 cup of chufa flour and mix well. I also added a cup of
chopped hickory-nut meats, but you can use almost any kind of
nuts. Dampen the hands and shape this stiff batter or dough into
little round balls the size of marbles, place well-separated on an ungreased cookie sheet, and bake in a 325° oven for about 20 minutes.
These will flatten on the bottom and will come out little brown
hemispheres of heavenliness. They can be eaten hot, warm, or cold,
and anyone who doesn't like them has crippled taste buds.

Recently my wife asked me if I could design a dessert that would
be good, unusual, and striking in appearance, to serve as a conversation piece at a New Year's dinner she was giving. I had been reading
an early American cookbook that was replete with recipes for boiled

puddings of many kinds, so I sent my culinary imagination in that direction. Not long ago I became interested in making meal from popcorn, finding it the best cornmeal I ever tasted, so I married this popcorn interest with my current chufa fad and came up with one of the best boiled puddings I have ever made.

Popcorn meal is no more than fine-ground popcorn that has been dry-popped, that is, popped without butter or oil. Always grind it in that ubiquitous electric blender, for other mills crush the grains before grinding them and rob the finished product of its attractive lightness. When reduced to a powder in a blender, popcorn meal is so light and fluffy that it will almost float away. A cupful of raw popcorn will make more than 2 quarts of finished meal.

My Chufa Pudding sounds like an incongruous mixture of ingredients, but it turns out to be a delectable combination. I opened a pint jar of canned wild blueberries, drained them thoroughly, then shook them with some dry flour until they were evenly coated. This is very important, for unfloured berries will dye the pudding an unattractive blue. In a mixing bowl I combined 1 cup of chufa flour, 2 cups popcorn meal, ½ cup of regular wheat flour, ½ cup of sugar, 1 teaspoon of salt, a level teaspoon of soda, and a cup of beef suet chopped to the size of rice grains. My butcher gladly gave me the suet when I ordered the meat for the dinner. In another bowl I beat 2 eggs until they were fluffy, then added this and a cup of buttermilk to the dry mixture. Next I carefully stirred in the floured berries, taking care not to break or mash them. A clean piece of muslin was dipped in hot water, wrung out, then spread inside a bowl and sprinkled with dry flour. The batter was spooned into the cloth and tied, not too tightly so the pudding would have room to swell, then plunged into rapidly boiling water and boiled for 2 hours.

I timed the cooking so the pudding would be just ready at dessert time and could be served hot. I lifted it from the boiling water, held it under cold running water for a few seconds, then peeled away the bag. It looked a bit small and lonely on its large round platter, so I decided it needed a more dramatic appearance. I had gathered a quantity of wintergreen plants bearing their bright red berries to use as decorations, and still had some unused ones on hand. I arranged these pretty little plants around the pudding and stuck a couple of heavily berried sprigs of wintergreen at jaunty angles in its side. Then I made a depression in the top of the pudding, poured in a tablespoonful of cognac, set it alight and bore my creation to the table in blazing triumph. The economical spherical shape of this pudding made it look small, but it very efficiently divided into eight adequate servings, and when eaten with a sauce of sweetened unwhipped cream, it easily lived up to its grand entrance.

41. Just How Good Are Wild Foods?

I KNOW a woman who has a modern kitchen so devoted to efficiency that an "office area" occupies a large portion of it. Here she keeps posted two charts, one showing the vitamin and mineral contents of all commonly used foods and the other showing the "minimum daily requirement" for such nutrients. Then there is a desk that has a small office adding machine on it. In planning her meals she consults the charts, then adds, subtracts, alters, and changes her menus until the books balance. She wouldn't touch wild foods with the tip of a cooking spoon, because their mineral and vitamin contents remain largely unknown, and these foods do not appear on her charts. Their makeup can't be fed into an adding machine, so to include them in her menus would merely mess up her bookkeeping.

The adding machine seems to be thriving on these mathematically balanced menus, but her family is slowly declining on this diet of digits, since their interest in food seems to lag by the day.

A chart showing the average minimum daily requirements of certain nutrients can be a valuable tool in planning menus, but, let's face it, such a chart really tells us very little about the nutritional needs of any particular individual at any particular time. Vitamin and mineral needs vary with age, sex, the state of the health, amount and kind of exercise and activity we indulge in, and many other factors too numerous to mention. Even taking large quantities of some vitamins can increase our need for others. Also, there may be a wide difference between the minimum daily requirements shown on the charts and the maximum amount our bodies can use to produce glowing health. Finally, there are wide individual differences in vitamin and mineral needs simply because some of us can assimilate these nutrients more efficiently than others can.

The chart figures that show the vitamin and mineral contents of certain foods are usually only averages of the amounts that have been found in large numbers of tests, but these amounts are apt to vary widely in individual tests. If some chart-smart friend tells you that carrots have a vitamin A value of 11,000 International Units per 100 grams, you are justified in asking such questions as: Which carrots? Where were they grown? How mature were they when harvested? How were they fertilized? How much sun and water did they receive during the growing period? How long were they stored before they were cooked and eaten? All these variables can have significant effects on the vitamin A content of carrots. Actually, in individual tests some samples of carrots have been found to have no significant vitamin A value whatever, while others have proved to have a vitamin A value of up to 50,000 International Units per 100 grams, which is very high indeed. Other vegetable evaluations vary just as widely, for the same reasons. So, while a chart can tell us the average mineral and vitamin content of almost any commonly used vegetable, it tells us very little about the nutritional value of the particular vegetable that is on our table.

Another limitation of such food charts is that they are usually incomplete. Ordinarily, they list only a few of the better-known vitamins and minerals, and this can give the impression that these are the only important nutrients, and that those not listed can be safely ignored. This is not true. A vitamin can be defined as "a chemical substance found in food that is essential to health," so all vitamins are essential by definition.

Certain vitamins may be omitted from some charts simply because the foods listed do not contain significant quantities of them. Others may be left out because there is seldom a deficiency of them in a normal diet. Some are neglected merely because the inclusion of every known vitamin and essential mineral would make the charts too long and complicated. Still others are left out because they are hard to detect in chemical tests and the amounts present in many foods have not been ascertained. Then there are some for which the amounts required by the human body are not known with any certainty. I'm sure that there are others that have not been discovered.

Nutrition is still a growing science, and it is certain that the future will reveal new vitamins just as important as those we already know.

Most charts showing the mineral values of foods will list calcium, iron, and potassium, but how many charts have you seen that list cobalt, copper, and iodine? And yet, these latter trace elements are just as important as those listed, and the deficiency diseases caused by their absence in our food can be just as devastating.

Are such charts then of no value? Far from it. The minimum daily requirement charts are extremely valuable to the makers, sellers, and advertisers of vitamin pills. They also help acquaint the layman with the names and natures of a few of the essential nutrients and give him a rough idea of the amounts of these nutrients required by most of us to keep functioning properly.

Even though the figures on the charts showing the amounts of nutrients in various foods are only rough averages, rather than absolute quantities, they can still be valuable references in planning your menus, if you allow for their limitations. When we look at a chart and see that spinach averages 8,100 International Units of vitamin A per serving, while cabbage averages only 130 I.U., we can be pretty certain that spinach is a better source of vitamin A than cabbage. And when we see that a serving of orange juice contains about 50 milligrams of ascorbic acid, while the same amount of apple juice contains only about 1 milligram, we know which juice to serve if we want to fortify our families with vitamin C. Such are the sensible uses of food charts. I am afraid that when my precisionist friend reads this she will no longer be my friend, so I must hasten to give her all the credit I can. At least she has furnished the perfect example of how not to use a food chart.

Now, having adequately warned you of the limitations of all food charts, I am going to present some of my own tables. These have the same limitations as other such charts. The first one, and the only one that represents any original research on my part, is the most limited of all. It shows the ascorbic acid, or vitamin C, content of 14 herbal materials in milligrams per 100 grams, the carotene, or provitamin A, content of 8 materials in International Units per 100 grams, and the protein content of 3 herbs in grams per 100 grams.

This was not a random exploration. Each herb listed was selected and tested because there was some reason to suspect the presence of the substances sought in the tests. Some of the best clues came from

ASCORBIC ACID, CAROTENE, AND PROTEIN CONTENT
OF CERTAIN SELECTED HERBS

Herbal Material	Water	Ascorbic acid mg/100 g	Pro-vitamin A I.U./100 g	Protein g/100 g
Locust Blossoms *	86%	30	—	—
Winter-Cress Buds *	84%	163	2015	—
Winter-Cress Leaves *	87%	152	5067	—
Catnip Leaves †	82%	83	—	—
Nettle Leaves †	84%	76	6566	6.9
Ground-Ivy Herb †	86%	55	—	—
Violet Leaves †	83%	210	8258	—
Violet Blossoms †	86%	150	—	—
Day Lily Buds *	87%	43	983	3.1
Boneset Herb †	75%	67	—	—
Highbush-Cranberry Fruit †	81%	100	2105	—
Dandelion Buds *	86%	30	800	3.1
Wild Spearmint †	82%	68	8575	—
Wild Strawberry Leaves †	67%	229	—	—

* The gathering and use as well as complete descriptions of these herbs will be found in my book, *Stalking the Wild Asparagus*, McKay, 1962.
† These herbs are described and directions for their use are given in this volume.

old herbals that were written hundreds of years before the term *vitamin* was coined. When one saw the same herb recommended by many different herbalists to cure symptoms that we now recognize as signs of vitamin deficiencies, it did not take a very brilliant mind to deduce that these plants might contain vitamins. Usually they did, and sometimes in astounding quantities.

Other clues came from the herbal wisdom of my Pennsylvania Dutch neighbors. Guided by taste, instinct, and the folklore handed down by their ancestors, these people seem able to select unerringly the herbs that will best correct the vitamin deficiencies in their diet. As I have mentioned, even small children correct their vitamin C shortage by chewing on catnip and eating raw violet blossoms, while their elders make strawberry-leaf tea and boneset tea and eat quantities of dandelion greens every spring.

In selecting the herbs that were to be tested for carotene, or pro-vitamin A, we had other clues. Carotene, which the body easily transforms into vitamin A, is a yellow coloring matter, and one can expect to find it in herbs that are yellow, orange, or green in color. We were not surprised to find rich vitamin A values in such dark-green leaves as those that come from winter-cress, nettle, violet, and wild spearmint plants. There are also good reasons for the blanks in that Vitamin A column. There are no yellow or green colors in locust and violet blossoms, so it was not thought worthwhile to test these materials for vitamin A. Catnip, ground-ivy, boneset, and wild strawberry leaves are probably all rich in vitamin A, but since these herbs are not actually eaten, but are usually taken in a hot-water infusion, this carotene content, no matter how rich, would be dissipated in the processing. Ascorbic acid, or vitamin C, is water soluble, and part of it will pass into hot-water infusions, but vitamin A is not water-soluble, but oil-soluble, and the amount that would pass into a hot-water infusion would cure no vitamin A deficiencies. It would not be honest to publish figures on the vitamin A content of these plants when this content is unusable. Winter-cress buds, day-lily buds, and dandelion buds gave disappointing yields of vitamin A despite the presence of yellow color. Apparently the yellow coloring matter in these buds is not carotene.

I had the flower buds of dandelions and day-lilies analyzed for protein, because I had a theory that the developing pollen material in these incipient flowers would prove a rich source of this important food. The theory died an unpleasant death. While both materials gave fair yields of protein, they were little if any richer in this food than comparable leaf materials. However, research that says a plain "No" to a pet theory is still good research.

I must confess that two of the materials in this table, locust blossoms and dandelion buds, were subjected to nutritional tests despite the fact that there was no clear indication that they were outstandingly nutritious in any way. I happen to be exceedingly fond of these two wild foods, and, frankly, I was looking for a better excuse than my own gastronomic delight for making myself such a pig over these wild delicacies.

Each spring, when the black locust trees that line the road to my house become covered with great pendent clusters of snowy white blooms, I have a feast, in fact several feasts. I gather these clusters, dip them in a fritter batter, and fry them to a golden brown. I sprinkle each fragrant Locust Fritter with a little orange juice, roll them in granulated sugar, and eat them while they're still piping hot. They are superb.

Even earlier in the spring, when the first dandelions bloom, I go after the finest food the dandelion produces. I dig out the plants, open them up, and from the very center I take the tiny, tender buds that intend to develop into future blossoms. They are almost snow-white on the outside, and if one is cut open it is seen to be pale-yellow inside from the developing blossom material. Just boiled a few minutes, then seasoned with salt and butter, these pale little buds make one of the most delicious vegetables I've ever tasted. The flavor and texture are both reminiscent of artichoke hearts, but Dandelion Buds are as far above artichoke hearts as artichokes are above turnip greens.

The analyses give little justification for overeating either of these delightful wild foods. Both yield fairly high values of vitamin C, the vitamin A value of dandelion buds is high enough to be of some slight significance in nutrition, and their 3.1 percent of protein is pretty high, but both these tasty foods make a poor showing when they appear in the same table with such nutritional giants as winter-cress, nettles, and violet leaves. I will continue to enjoy these two delicacies each spring, but I'm afraid that hereafter I must admit that eating them is pure self-indulgence, rather than a prudent measure to protect my health.

Despite the limited scope of this research, we struck nutritional gold at several points. Violet leaves proved to have an almost unbelievably high ascorbic acid content, but they were tested, retested, then tested again with a fresh supply of leaves, and we could only come to the conclusion that this rich vitamin C value is really there. This is more than 4½ times the vitamin C value of an equal weight of oranges, which we usually consider to be a very rich source of this protective vitamin. A search through the U.S. Department of Agriculture's comprehensive work, *The Composition of Foods*, reveals that the violet leaf is far richer in vitamin C than any leafy vegetable they list. It is also an excellent source of carotene, or provitamin A. As explained in the chapter on this herb, violet greens should be eaten in moderation or mixed with other greens, but even a moderate amount of this vitamin-rich herb can furnish a tremendous amount of nutrition.

Winter-cress, dandelion greens, nettle greens, and curled dock are all in season at the same time that violet leaves are at their best. I have tried cooking all these greens in many combinations, and find them all palatable. All five mixed together, boiled and seasoned with a little crisp bacon and finely chopped raw onion, make a delicious

blend of Mixed Greens, and this is probably one of the most nutritious vegetable dishes that can be devised. Don't overlook those
violet blossoms. A few of them scattered over a tossed salad not only
make a beautiful garnish, but they also add a pleasant flavor and
furnish real nutrition. Although not as vitamin-packed as the leaves,
the fragrant blossoms are still three times as rich in vitamin C as an
equal amount of orange juice. No wonder that vitamin-C-starved
children develop a taste for violet blossoms. Another nutritious and
tasty addition to that tossed salad would be some fine-chopped wild
spearmint. This herb is also an excellent source of vitamin C and
an even better source of vitamin A. There is health among the herbs
if you know how to find it.

The reason for assaying the protein content of nettles was that I
had read a report from Germany, dating from First World War days,
on the use of dried nettles in feeding livestock. The report stated
that this material was more nutritious than any kind of grain and
that it apparently had a higher protein content than linseed oil cake.
I simply didn't believe this, for linseed oil cake is considered a protein concentrate, with an average protein content of about 35 percent. Again I was wrong, but this time in a very pleasing way. That
6.9 percent of protein shown for green nettles is an amazing yield
for a green, leafy material, higher than that of any leafy vegetable in
the aforementioned *Composition of Foods*. Calculated on a dry-
weight basis, this gives a protein value of about 42 percent, so that
German report actually understated the nutritional value of dried
nettle leaves. When one sees this unprecedented yield of protein in
a very palatable green vegetable that is also an excellent source of vitamins A and C, then one knows that here is a nutritional find that is
going to be hard to excel. This may well be the single most important
discovery made in this series of food tests.

Winter-cress, *Barbarea vulgaris*, is a member of the mustard family and is often called "wild mustard" by those farmers whose fields
it infests. It has the advantage of being available during the winter
and very early spring, growing rapidly during any warm spell. From
New York southward, one can usually pick a mess of winter-cress
greens any time the ground is not covered by snow. As the tables
show, winter-cress greens have three times the vitamin C value of an
equal weight of orange juice and are an excellent source of vitamin
A. They are cooked and served like spinach. In late spring the clus-

ters of unopened buds may be gathered and cooked like broccoli, to which this plant is closely related. The buds have an even higher vitamin C content than the leaves, but are only about half as rich in vitamin A.

The chief value of such herbs as ground-ivy and the fruit of the highbush-cranberry or guelder-rose is that their rather rich vitamin C content is available during the winter months. Formerly, before citrus fruits were commonly imported by northern countries, and before the development of bottled, canned, and frozen foods, almost everyone in the northern regions suffered more or less vitamin C deficiency in the wintertime. Scurvy was almost epidemic in late winter. Ground-ivy and the fruit of the guelder-rose were the wonder drugs of that day, seemingly magically healing all those multiple symptoms that are the result of vitamin C deficiency. Boneset is chiefly valuable as a bitter tonic, and it may have as-yet-undiscovered beneficial drugs, but part of its value, too, may have lain in its fairly rich vitamin C content.

That wild strawberry leaves were one of the richest natural sources of vitamin C was another of our important discoveries. Like ground-ivy, the strawberry is winter-hardy and keeps producing a few green leaves even in the dead of winter, when other natural sources of vitamin C are hard to come by.

Strawberry leaves can be eaten in emergencies, but the taste and texture are nothing to go into ecstasies about. The best way to capture this almost unheard-of high vitamin C content is in a Strawberry Leaf Extract. Fill your blender jar with freshly picked strawberry leaves, cover with water, and blend at slow speed just until the leaves are cut fine, not until they are beaten to a pulp. Put this soup in a saucepan, bring just to a boil, then simmer for 15 minutes. Allow the chopped leaves to stand in the cooking water until next day, then strain. By this time the greater part of that rich vitamin C content will have passed into the water. This watery extract is very mild in flavor, with a slight fragrance of roses. I have not had samples of the extract tested, but would wager that it is richer in vitamin C than the finest orange juice. We use this vitamin-rich extract to dilute frozen concentrated juices, or we mix it with a little cider vinegar and sweeten it with honey to taste, and it makes a very tasty breakfast beverage.

I live far out in the country and have acres of wild strawberries

	water: percentage	food energy: calories/100 g	protein: g/100 g	carbohydrates: g/100g total	carbohydrates: g/100g fiber	ash: g/100g	calcium: mg/100 g	phosphorus: mg/100g	iron: mg/100 g	potassium: mg/100 g	vitamin A: I.U./100 g	ascorbic acid: mg/100g
WILD VEGETABLE												
Green Amaranth *	86.9	36	3.5	6.5	1.3	2.6	267	67	3.9	411	6100	80
Wild Asparagus *	91.7	26	2.5	5.0	0.7	0.6	22	62	1.0	278	900	33
Chicory Greens *	92.8	20	1.8	3.8	0.8	1.3	86	40	0.9	420	4000	22
Dandelion Greens *	85.6	45	2.7	9.2	1.6	1.8	187	66	3.1	397	14000	35
Lamb's-Quarters *	84.3	43	4.2	7.3	2.1	3.4	309	72	1.2	—	11600	80
Poke Shoots *	91.6	23	2.6	3.7	—	1.7	53	44	1.7	—	8700	136
Purslane *	92.5	21	1.7	3.8	0.9	1.6	103	39	3.5	—	2500	25
Watercress *	93.3	19	2.2	3.0	0.7	1.2	151	54	1.7	282	4900	79
Curled Dock †	90.9	28	2.1	5.6	0.8	1.1	66	41	1.6	338	12900	119

Some commonly eaten domestic green vegetables for comparison

	water: percentage	food energy: calories/100 g	protein: g/100 g	carbohydrates: g/100g total	carbohydrates: g/100g fiber	ash: g/100g	calcium: mg/100 g	phosphorus: mg/100g	iron: mg/100 g	potassium: mg/100 g	vitamin A: I.U./100 g	ascorbic acid: mg/100g
GARDEN VEGETABLE												
Cabbage	92.4	24	1.3	5.4	0.8	0.7	49	29	0.4	233	130	51
Celery	94.1	17	0.9	3.9	0.6	1.0	39	28	0.3	341	240	9
Endive	93.1	20	1.7	4.1	0.9	1.0	81	54	1.7	294	3300	10
Iceberg Lettuce	95.5	13	0.9	2.9	0.5	0.6	20	22	0.5	175	330	6
Leaf Lettuce	94.0	18	1.3	3.5	0.7	0.9	68	25	1.4	264	1900	18
Green Onions	89.4	36	1.5	8.2	1.2	0.7	51	39	1.0	231	2000	32
Green Peppers	93.4	22	1.2	4.8	1.4	0.4	9	22	0.7	213	420	128
Spinach	90.7	26	3.2	4.3	0.6	1.5	93	51	3.1	470	8100	51
Swiss Chard	91.1	25	2.4	4.6	0.8	1.6	88	39	3.2	550	6500	32

* Description and directions for use of these wild foods given in *Stalking the Wild Asparagus*, McKay, 1962.

† This herb described and directions given for its use in this volume.

	water: percentage	food energy: calories/100 g	protein: g/100 g	carbohydrates: g/100 g total	carbohydrates: g/100 g fiber	ash: g/100 g	calcium: mg/100 g	phosphorus: mg/100 g	iron: mg/100 g	potassium: mg/100 g	vitamin A: I.U./100 g	ascorbic acid: mg/100 g
WILD FRUIT												
Blackberries *	85.4	58	1.2	12.9	4.1	.5	32	19	0.9	170	200	21
Blueberries *	83.2	62	0.7	15.3	1.5	.3	15	13	1.0	60	40	6
Elderberries *	93.1	20	1.7	4.1	0.9	1.0	81	54	1.7	294	3300	10
Ground Cherries *	85.4	53	1.9	11.2	2.8	.8	9	40	1.0	—	720	11
Red Haws †	75.8	87	2.0	20.8	2.1	.8	—	—	—	—	—	—
Wild Persimmons *	64.4	127	0.8	33.5	1.5	.9	27	26	2.5	310	—	66
Prickly Pears §	88.0	42	0.5	10.9	1.6	.5	20	28	0.3	166	60	22
Black Raspberries *	80.8	73	1.5	15.7	5.1	.6	30	22	0.9	199	trace	18
Red Raspberries *	84.2	57	1.2	13.6	3.0	.5	22	22	0.9	168	130	25
Some commonly eaten domestic fruits for comparison												
ORCHARD FRUIT												
Apples	84.4	58	0.2	14.5	1.0	.3	7	10	0.3	110	90	4
Oranges	86.0	49	1.0	12.2	0.5	.6	41	20	0.4	200	200	50
Peaches	89.1	38	0.6	9.7	0.6	.5	9	19	0.5	202	1330	7
Pears	83.2	61	0.7	15.3	1.4	.4	8	11	0.3	130	20	4
Japanese Persimmons	78.6	77	0.7	19.7	1.6	.6	6	26	0.3	174	2710	11
Tomatoes	93.5	22	1.1	4.7	0.5	.5	13	27	0.5	244	900	23
Gooseberries	88.9	39	0.8	9.7	1.9	.4	18	15	0.5	155	290	33

— (Blanks with dashes) means there are no data available. The food in question may contain this nutrient, indeed it may be rich in it, but the quantity has never been ascertained.

* Descriptions and directions for using these fruits found in *Stalking the Wild Asparagus*, McKay, 1962.

† Description and directions for using this fruit found in this volume.

§ Description and directions for using this fruit found in *Stalking the Blue-Eyed Scallop*, McKay, 1964.

practically at my doorstep, and, since I can make this extract any time I want it, I seldom make a large quantity at a time. However, for those not so happily situated, I have worked out a method of freezing Strawberry Leaf Extract. Make it just as directed above, adding 2 tablespoons of cider vinegar, or 2 tablespoons of lemon juice if you prefer it, to each pint of extract, then pour it into containers and freeze it. Be sure to add the lemon juice or vinegar before freezing, for this acid is necessary to prevent enzymes from destroying the vitamin C content. When it is to be used, thaw at room temperature, then sweeten with honey to taste.

Now, let's look at the composition of some of the other wild fruits and vegetables that I have mentioned in this book or in previous works. The figures in the following tables were taken from a book called *Composition of Foods*, Agricultural Handbook No. 8, published by the Agricultural Research services of the United States Department of Agriculture.

Guests at my "wild parties" often ask me if it is possible to get the vitamins, minerals, and other nutritional elements one needs from wild food. Well, here is the answer, in these charts. Looking first at the vegetable chart, one sees that the wild vegetables are consistently ahead of their domestic counterparts in all categories. Dandelion greens, curled dock and lamb's-quarters (pigweed) all give higher yields of vitamin A than any other leafy vegetables listed in *Composition of Foods*. Both green amaranth and purslane have higher iron content than any other green vegetable listed except parsley, which has a whopping 6.2 milligrams per 100 grams. Did you ever eat 100 grams (about 3½ ounces, or nearly ¼ pound) of parsley at one sitting? I never did, although I have often eaten that much amaranth and purslane. That 3.5 milligrams of iron in purslane is a startling amount in a plant that is 92.5 percent water.

Both amaranth and purslane are among the most common of all weeds, being found in disturbed ground everywhere. I doubt that there is a single county between Canada and Mexico, and between the Atlantic and the Pacific, where these weeds cannot be found. Millions of tons of these outstandingly nutritious vegetables go to waste every year, with not more than a tiny fraction of one percent of the total being eaten. And yet, both these plants can be made into very palatable dishes that would grace the most refined table in the land.

Look again at that lowly lawn weed, the dandelion. It is an excellent source of calcium and potassium, and the best known source of vitamin A among the green vegetables. And yet, we spend millions on herbicides to kill the dandelions in our lawns, while we pay millions more for diet supplements to give ourselves the vitamins and minerals that the dandelion could easily furnish. Beyond that, the dandelion furnishes some of the most palatable of all green vegetables, the favorite greens of thousands of country people who eat them every spring with an avidity that resembles a religious rite.

Lamb's-quarters or pigweed, *Chenopodium album*, is a close relative of garden spinach, and the chart shows that it is by far the better plant of the two. It is richer in vitamin C, far richer in vitamin A, and, while not quite as rich as spinach in iron and potassium, it is still a good source of these important minerals. But the area where lamb's-quarters really excels is as a source of calcium. Those 309 milligrams of calcium per 100 grams make this the richest source of calcium found among the green leafy vegetables listed in the *Composition of Foods*, and green amaranth is the second richest vegetable source, with turnip greens a poor third. Lamb's-quarters is also a very common weed, being found in cultivated ground from border to border and coast to coast, and it can usually be found in just the right stage for eating from late spring until frost.

Poke shoots and greens, and dock greens are all exceedingly nutritious vegetables, excellent sources of vitamins A and C, that offer splendid yields of several essential minerals. I have always considered wild watercress a very nutritious salad green, and so it is when compared to lettuce, cabbage, and celery, but placed in a chart among such super-nutritious greens as amaranth, dandelion, lamb's-quarters, poke shoots, and curled dock, it looks so puny as to seem hardly worth the eating.

Yes, it is possible to get enough vitamins and minerals from wild foods to maintain health; in fact, it would be difficult to become undernourished if we would only eat the delicious wild herbs and vegetables that grow all about us.

Now, let us look at the chart showing the nutritional value of some of the fruits, wild and tame. The wild fruits do not come away trailing quite as many clouds of glory as do the wild vegetables, but their nutritional value is nothing to sneer at. Look carefully at that chart and you will see that in every desirable category it is a wild fruit that takes the prize.

The common native persimmon, found growing wild, often in great but neglected abundance, from New York to Florida and west to the Great Plains, runs away with most of the blue ribbons, being first in food energy, carbohydrates, iron, potassium, and ascorbic acid, a wonderfully nutritious fruit. When tree-ripened to perfection, the persimmon is one of the tastiest of all fruits, as well as being one of the most nutritious, and in the hands of a clever cook this luscious wild fruit can be transformed into some of the most palatable dishes that ever came to the table.

The wild black elderberry, which goes to waste by the thousands of tons every year, comes in a close second, being first in calcium and vitamin A and very rich in iron and potassium. This wild fruit grows in great abundance along fencerows, roadsides, and stream valleys throughout the eastern half of our country, and has been naturalized on the West Coast. Unlike many wild fruits, the elderberry is not tedious to gather. The berries are borne in great umbels, or cymes, that seem to beg to be broken off and made into fine jams, jellies, fruit sauces, pies, and spicy elderberry wine. The other wild fruits in the list don't come off quite as well as the elderberry and persimmon, but they do very well when compared with the domestic fruits.

Finally, let us examine a little-known class of wild foods, the edible seaweeds. Not much is known for certain about them, and the few figures in this little chart were taken from that same book, *Composition of Foods*, from which this chapter has drawn so freely. The sea is the final repository of all the essential minerals that have been leached from the land through the ages, and every element is found in sea water. We naturally expect the plants that grow in this mineral-rich environment to be nutritious, and, judging from the little this chart tells us about them, they do not disappoint us.

This chart immediately shows us that seaweeds are generally much richer in calcium than land plants, and when it comes to potassium, the land plants are not even in the running. The one example given of iron content shows that seaweed is far ahead of any land-grown vegetable we know, as a source of this important mineral. But the most important benefits that seaweeds can contribute to our health are not shown on this chart.

The ocean is not just water, but a marvelously complex liquid,

KNOWN CONSTITUENTS OF SOME EDIBLE SEAWEEDS

	water: percentage	fat: g/100 g	fiber: g/100 g	ash: g/100 g	calcium: mg/100 g	phosphorus: mg/100 g	iron: mg/100 g	sodium: mg/100 g	potassium: mg/100 g
Dulse	16.6	3.2	1.2	22.4	296	267	—	2085	8060
Irish Moss	19.2	1.8	2.1	17.6	885	157	—	2892	2844
Edible Kelp	21.9	1.1	6.8	22.8	1093	240	8.9	3007	5273
Laver	17.0	0.6	3.5	11.0	—	—	—	—	—

containing, in solution, all the essential minerals and trace elements the human body needs for life and health. Plants growing in this mineral richness take up these elements and convert them into usable, organic form. Our bodies need dozens of these essential minerals and trace elements. Some are needed only in minute quantities, it is true, but their absence can keep our glands and organs from functioning properly, and we may sicken, or even die, from the lack of a microscopic amount of some obscure mineral. Land plants grown in mineral-starved soils cannot provide these nutrients, but seaweed can. Your thyroid needs iodine; both the parathyroid and the pancreas need cobalt and nickel; the gonads require iron; the anterior pituitary gland needs manganese; the posterior pituitary needs chlorine, and other glands, organs, and even the individual cells of our bodies require many other minerals. If we fail to furnish our bodies with an adequate supply of even one of these minerals, we imperil our health. The edible seaweeds could give us an abundant supply of all the minerals we need, if we would only learn to eat them.

I have gathered and experimented with all four of the seaweeds listed in this chart, and have managed to concoct some perfectly edible, and even palatable, dishes from all of them. The methods and recipes will be found in my book *Stalking the Blue-Eyed Scallop*. In Nova Scotia and New Brunswick, dulse is gathered, dried, and sold in the grocery stores. The local people eat this dried seaweed as a relish with other foods, or as a pleasant nibble or between-meals snack. This is not consciously done as a health measure, for many of these people never heard of trace minerals. They eat dulse purely because they like it. While traveling in these provinces I acquired a taste for dulse, and now I am never without a supply of this tasty tidbit.

If we could spread this dulse-chewing habit throughout our land it would be one of the greatest public-health services ever performed. Goiter would disappear, a host of other mineral deficiency diseases would no longer endanger our health and lives, and millions of people would be healthier than they now are. These edible seaweeds may yet prove to be the most important healthful herbs mentioned in this book.

The most astonishing thing to be learned from all these charts is not the nutritional discoveries, important as they are. In this study, the thing that surprised and saddened me was to discover just how little this super-scientific age knows about the wild plants that cover our earth and grow beneath our seas. In a few areas our knowledge is extensive. The botanists and taxonomists have done their work well. The job of discovering, collecting, describing, classifying, and naming the wild plants is almost finished, and new discoveries in this field are becoming increasingly rare. It is in the use of these wild plants that we are still abysmally ignorant. The chemical, medicinal, nutritional, and gastronomic investigation of wild plants has hardly begun. Who says there are no frontiers left? The student who longs for an unknown field to explore need go no farther than the nearest vacant lot.

As a result of this meager little study, a few generalizations can safely be made. On the whole, it seems that edible wild plants are considerably more nutritious than the domestic plants that we commonly eat. Certainly there are many wild plants that could, with great profit to our health and well-being, be added to our daily diet. Ridiculous as it sounds, we might be better off nutritionally if we threw away the crops that we so laboriously raise in our fields and gardens and ate the weeds that grow with no encouragement from us—indeed they grow despite all our strenuous efforts to eradicate them. Health-food enthusiasts may discover that the finest health-food stores are the woods and fields, the roadsides and seashores, yes, and even that patch of weeds in the corner of the garden. And best of all, the merchandise in all these stores is free.

But wild foods are not only good for you, they are good. They can bring us new taste thrills, exotic and delicious flavors, and add to the joy of eating. I have proved in my own kitchen that hundreds of wild foods can be made into dishes that will delight the most particular gourmet, and my wild parties have achieved a measure of fame.

Gathering and using wild foods is my hobby, and I long suspected that my preference for the flavors of wild foods was psychogenic in origin. I was afraid that my taste had been influenced by the pleasure this activity brought me, and explained the enjoyment of my guests by thinking that my enthusiasm might be a bit contagious. But the explanation is much simpler than I thought. As a result of this study I have concluded that the reason wild foods taste better is that they are better. It's as simple as that.

42. Capturing Wild Perfumes

OUR PREHISTORIC ANCESTORS discovered and used the natural fragrances found in many wild plants. Some primitive housewife may have covered the rough, dirt floor of her cave or hut with the stalks and leaves of calamus,* intending merely to make it more comfortable to sit and lie on, and discovered that this fragrant plant filled her habitation with an interesting spicy aroma that dispelled the general smelliness that had prevailed there before. Her mate was entranced by the new smell, and evn the neighbor men trotted over for a whiff, filling her pretty little head with the idea that maybe good smells could be used to attract men.

While scrubbing the flat stone on which she served her mate's food, in the stream that served as her dishpan, she may have pulled a handful of mint to use as a dishtowel, and discovered that the stale, greasy odor, that would have been a feature of such porous dishes in a soapless culture, was replaced by a clean, appetizing aroma. Gathering soft foliage to make the family couch more comfortable, she must have included sweet-smelling grasses, aromatic spruce boughs, sweet fern leaves, wild lavender, and other fragrant plants, and discovered that they not only replaced the ugly odor of the animal skins and covered the bed with a sweet, sleep-inducing aroma, but found that this smell also made her combative mate more amiable.

Primitive peoples had to have a more acute sense of smell than we do, for they used their noses to seek and identify certain plants and

---

* Discussed in greater detail in *Stalking the Wild Asparagus*.

foods, to test the environment, to scent danger, and for many other survival purposes.

We know that prehistoric man must have used perfume, because in the earliest writings of recorded history, those of the Egyptians, Hebrews, Babylonians, Assyrians, and Chinese, we find that perfumery is already a sophisticated and highly developed art. Today, modern science has entered the field of scent in a big way. We have developed synthetic scents that rival those of nature, and have found how to combine them with fixatives, diffusers, and preservatives and sell them through advertisements that would be salacious if they were not so ridiculous. The use of manufactured perfumes has become universal, and millions of gallons are sold annually.

However, I don't think that man, with all his talent and skill, has actually surpassed nature as a maker of sweet scents. Does the very finest rose perfume smell quite as sweet as a newly blown rose, and does the most expensive product of the perfumer's art really surpass the fragrance of a freshly opened lily of the valley? When I try making scents of naturally fragrant materials I don't try to make them smell like expensive perfumes, but attempt to capture, unspoiled, the pure, natural fragrances with which nature has endowed certain plant materials.

The best way to assure yourself of a perfectly natural, unchanged scent is to use the fragrant materials that nature produces in such abundance just as you find them, with no preparation whatever. Once, when a group of journalists had been invited to my house for a wild dinner, I decided to give their olfactory, as well as their gustatory, senses a feast. Over my wife's strenuous objections, I covered the entrance hall floor with freshly cut calamus leaves, so my guests were greeted by its spicy, amorous aroma. From beside a nearby stream I gathered about a half-bushel of fresh mint, and made a path of the plants on the dining-room floor from the entrance door to the table. As the guests walked in to take their places, the appetizing odor of fresh mint, entirely different from the smell of peppermint oil or spearmint flavoring, permeated the room without dominating the equally appetizing smells of the food. I had prepared sassafras * tea for the dinner, and as I boiled these fragrant roots in the kitchen their ambrosial bouquet filled that room and spilled over into the

---

* Discussed in greater detail in *Stalking the Wild Asparagus*.

rest of the house, blending with the other natural perfumes that gladdened the air.

It would be impossible to scent a house to this extent with commercial perfumes and still remain within the bounds of good taste, but, because these were natural fragrances, unalloyed with synthetics, fixatives, diffusers, animal perfumes, or alcohol, they were perfectly acceptable, and my guests, without exception, found this feast of aromas delightful. These blended smells served as olfactory hors d'oeuvres, giving a teasing pretaste of the dinner to come. The guests were delighted to find calamus hearts in the salad, sassafras in the herb tea, and candied mint leaves passed after dinner, which they instantly recognized as the flavor side of the aromas that had titillated their noses.

These perfectly natural fragrances can also be used to perfume the clothes one wears. We are all familiar with sachets, those dainty little bags containing dried lavender flowers, dried rose petals, or mixtures of spices, that our grandmothers used to bury among their clothes to give them a delightful aroma. The same principle can be used to perfume clothes with wild fragrances that can't be imitated by commercial perfumers. And you don't have to settle for that grandmotherly smell of lavender and old lace which the word *sachet* brings to most memories. I am addicted to bulky, loud-patterned, Scandinavian wool sweaters, but I detest the odor of commercial moth repellents, so I've worked out a way to protect these treasures with a natural repellent that is fragrant. I make a mixture of 1 pound of pine needles, 1 ounce of cedar shavings, and about ½ ounce of shavings from the root of sassafras. The needles from Western piñon pine are best, but you can use the foliage from any fragrant pine; let your nose be your guide. These quantities can be tampered with if you wish to create your own original mixture, but be careful with those cedar chips and sassafras, for these odors tend to dominate the compound if used too freely. I have found that I can even use freshly cut pine needles, if I scatter them loosely, without starting mold or rot. Line a drawer with paper, sprinkle in the mixture and cover with a thickness of cloth (a piece from an old sheet will do), fastening the cloth firmly in place with thumbtacks. Store your woolens on top and they will not only be protected from depredations of moths, but will come out with a clean, masculine fragrance that fairly shouts of forests, mountains, and the great manly outdoors.

The girls can get into the act, too, for not all wild fragrances are so masculine. In our section of Pennsylvania, and on through the mountains to Georgia, grows a wildflower that is commonly known as deertongue, mountain-lettuce, or lettuce-saxifrage. Its Latin name is *Saxifraga micranthidifolia*, if anybody cares. It grows in swampy places and along cool mountain streams, appearing early in the spring as a rosette of leaves four to ten inches long, shaped like a deer's tongue, sharply toothed on the margins. (The local hillbillies, and my own family, gather these first early leaves while they are tender and cook them with bacon and a bit of sour cream and find it a very good dish. You can cook these early leaves by any of the recipes given for cooking wild lettuce (see page 40).) Later on, an almost naked flower scape rises from the center of the rosette of leaves and becomes two to three feet high, bearing a panicle of small white flowers. If the leaves are gathered about the time the plant flowers, and dried by spreading them on papers in a warm room, they develop an aroma that slightly resembles the fragrance of vanilla. My wife uses these sweet-smelling leaves to line the drawer in which she keeps her sweaters, and when she wears a sweater perfumed by this plant she smells sweet enough to eat.

Calamus, or sweet flag, grows throughout the United States and around the world in the North Temperate Zone. It looks like a diminutive cat-tail without the tail, or an overgrown wild iris without the iris, except that the color of the sword-shaped leaves is a lighter green, with more yellow in its makeup, than the color of either of the aforementioned plants. It grows in marshes and low meadows and at pondsides, in great patches, the individual plants standing about three feet high. The lower stems and the underground rhizomes have a spicy, pungent, and fascinating aroma that is very persistent, and is still quite pronounced when the materials are dried. The lower stems or the rhizomes, or both, can be dried in a warm room, then cut into fairly fine pieces and used to make a sweet-smelling drawer lining or put into small porous bags to be hung in the clothes closet. They will give protection from moths and also give the clothes a pleasant and exciting smell. I hereby disclaim all responsibility for anything that may happen to you while wearing calamus-scented clothing, however, since the aroma of this plant has long been thought to be somewhat aphrodisiac.

There are those who prefer to capture these wild fragrances in liquid perfumes that can be stored in bottles or vials. This is a wonderful way of preserving the fragrance of wild flowers so that you can bring summer right back into your house during a winter blizzard merely by uncorking a vial. The equipment for making this natural perfume can be easily assembled in any household. The process is so simple that even a child can do it. All you need is a glass jar with a tight-fitting lid, some absorbent cotton, and some sweet oil, which is no more than highly refined olive oil that can be purchased in any drugstore. Fill the jar two-thirds full of fragrant flowers, saturate the cotton in sweet oil, just to the point where it will not drip, spread the cotton over the flowers, cover the jar, and let it sit in the sun all day. Next day, empty out the flowers and refill the jar with fresh ones. Continue to do this as long as the season lasts for the flowers you are using. By the end of the season, the oil in the cotton will be highly charged with exactly the same fragrance that arose from the fresh flower, and it can be squeezed into a vial or bottle. It is best kept in the refrigerator so that the oil won't become rancid. Be sure that you use a *glass* jar for this operation. A plastic container will not do, for it will make your product smell just like a plastic container, and it would be hard for me to think of anything that smells worse.

Using the above method you can make your own original perfume from any fragrance you happen to like. The blossoms from some flowering trees work exceedingly well. The magnolia and the sweet bay both make lazy, Southern fragrances that are very alluring. Mimosa blooms give a heavy, sweet, almost Oriental aroma that hints of mystery. Some species of wild rose have clean, virginal fragrances. If you want to go further afield for an exclusive perfume that every Jane and Jill won't be wearing, try making some scent from the clusters of purplish-brown blooms of the groundnut * (*Apios americana*), which grows as a thin, trailing vine in low grounds throughout the eastern half of the United States. These blossoms have a rich, heady fragrance, and not every woman can live up to such a scent, but if you are daring, try it. Or maybe you would prefer the sweet, schoolgirlish fragrance of the white, clustered blossoms of the black locust (*Robinia pseudo-acacia*). These blossoms are abundant every spring wherever this common tree grows, so you will have no trouble finding the material.

* Discussed in greater detail in *Stalking the Wild Asparagus*.

You are not limited to the scents of flowers while using this method of concentrating natural fragrances. Almost any scent that happens to please your fancy can be captured in this way. A piece of aromatic cedar (*Juniperus virginiana*) can be reduced to shavings, either on the jointer at the lumberyard where you buy it, or at home with a hand plane. These shavings can be placed in the jar instead of flowers, and you will not have to change them often, for this aroma is very persistent. It imbues the oil in the cotton with an aromatic, cedar-chest fragrance. Shavings made in the same way from the root-wood of sassafras can be used in the same way. Using the lower stems and rhizomes of calamus, you can make an exciting perfume that is reputed to turn timid men into satyrs. A very interesting perfume can be made by placing a dozen or two papaw * fruits in a jar and covering them with the oiled cotton until the fruits are ripened to your taste. This is a heavy, sweet, almost cloying scent that is effective when used with extreme discretion.

How shall we use the oil once we have made it? If you are interested enough to explore the whole perfumer's art you can learn to mix the oil with alcohol and add small quantities of those interesting animal perfumes that serve as fixatives, diffusers, and modifiers. These are ambergris, musk, castor, and civet, all unbelievably expensive. Ambergris is a calculus, or pathological secretion, from a sick sperm whale. It is recovered from the intestines of the whale by professional whalers, or found floating on the sea or cast up on the beach by lucky beachcombers. Musk is from the dried glands of a certain species of Asiatic deer. Castor is a scent gland recovered by trappers from the Canadian or Russian beaver. Civet is a soft, fatty substance secreted by the glands of a small animal of Abyssinia.

My own experiments with blending the fragrant oil from my glass jar with exotic ingredients that were supposed to improve it have been very disappointing. Each new ingredient that I added made the scented oil smell less like the natural fragrance from which it was derived and more like a commercial, manufactured product. I finally decided it would be better to use the oil as it is squeezed from the cotton, and let it take care of its own diffusion, fixation, and modification. A dab or two of the pure scented oil behind the ears, or a drop or two combed through the hair, diffuses a subtle, delightful odor that will give a woman the aura of a field of fragrant wildflowers rather than that of a cosmetic counter.

Glossary

IN THIS BOOK I have tried to avoid as much technical jargon as possible, but I soon saw that the total circumvention of all specialized vocabulary would make the descriptions of the plants and their properties too wordy. Reluctantly, I decided to include a short glossary defining only those technical terms that I couldn't evade. The list included here was derived by having my editor, my wife, and several long-suffering friends read the manuscript and submit lists of words that I had used which they thought needed further clarification. The result is a hodge-podge of medical, herbal, botanical, and even a few horticultural and culinary terms, arranged in alphabetical order, with no attempt to separate them into their various categories. This glossary, since it is purposely limited to as few terms as such subject matter will permit, would be of no use whatever in studying other works on herbs, botany, or any of the other sciences I dip into, but was designed solely to help you understand any unfamiliar term you may encounter in this book.

Air layering: A means of propagating desirable strains of plants by first scarring a limb, then wrapping it in soil, sphagnum moss, or some other rooting medium, and allowing roots to grow in this bandage. The branch is then severed between the air layer and the trunk, and planted. It becomes an independent plant with all the characteristics of the parent tree.

Alterative: An old-fashioned medical term meaning a medicine that cures an illness by gradually restoring general bodily health.

Antibiotic: An organic chemical substance, derived from living things, that will work selectively against harmful microorganisms. The term and the explanation are new, but that such substances could cure disease has been known to primitive herbalists for thousands of years.

Antipyretic: Any medicine for checking or preventing fever. Also called *febrifuge* and *refrigerant.*

Antiscorbutic: A food or medicine that can prevent or cure scurvy. Any plant that contains significant amounts of vitamin C (and most fresh green plants do contain this vitamin) is an antiscorbutic.

Antiseptic: A substance that will destroy the microorganisms that cause infection.

Antispasmodic: A relaxant that will relieve or prevent the involuntary contractions that appear in epilepsy, spastic paralysis, painful menstruation, or even the "charley horses" that afflict athletes.

Aperient: A mild and gentle-acting laxative.

Aromatic: A plant, drug, or medicine with a spicy scent and pungent but pleasing taste. Such fragrance and flavor can sometimes revive the faint, elevate the depressed, and set a despairing patient on the road to recovery.

Astringent: Any substance that causes tissue to shrink or pucker. Alum is a familiar astringent.

Beverages and bottles: Home-made beverages will keep better if sealed in amber or green glass bottles than if clear glass is used. Clear glass admits too much light, which debases the flavor of most beverages, giving them a "skunky" taste. Bottles should be sealed with crown caps, which are exactly like the caps on most soda bottles except for the printed advertising matter. These caps must be put on with a bottle capper. Both caps and capper can be purchased at most hardware stores.

Calculus: Not higher math, but in this case a stone that forms in some bodily organ because of a diseased condition. Kidney stones, gallstones, and bladder stones are examples of calculi.

Calmative: An old herbalist's term for any plant or medicine that seems to soothe the patient's central nervous system and allow him to rest quietly.

Cambium: The layer of tender, forming cells between the bark and the trunk of a tree. It is gorged with rich sap containing sugars and starches, and the cambium from some trees makes good and nutritious food.

Carminative: An herb or tidbit that will discourage the formation of gas after eating, or help expel gas that has already formed.

Catkin: A downy or scaly spike of flowers produced by certain plants and trees. The "pussy" on a willow is an example. On some trees, catkins are called "aments."

Cellulose: The substance that forms the walls of most plant cells. This is the woody part of a tree. Cellulose is a perfectly good carbohydrate, but unfortunately human beings can't digest it.

Chemurgic: Adjective pertaining to that branch of chemistry that deals with the uses of organic raw materials from plants and animals.

Corm: The enlarged, fleshy base of certain plants, bulb-shaped but solid, usually starchy, and often edible. The turnip and the radish are examples of corms.

Counterirritant: A substance that causes irritation, or mild pain, on the body's surface in order to relieve a deeper and more acute pain. This actually works. The minor surface pain created by the counterirritant ties up the sensory nerves so the deeper pain can't get through to the brain with its message of suffering. The deeper pain is still there, but you are no longer aware of it. It is something like trying to impart terrible news by telephone, only to find the party line tied up by someone who wants to whine about very minor complaints.

Cystitis: An infection of the urinary tract.

Deobstruent: An herb or medicine that has the power to clear obstructions from the natural ducts of the body.

Demulcent: A substance that is soothing to the gastrointestinal tract. Slippery elm and mallow, because of their mucilaginous natures, are both excellent demulcents.

Diaphoretic: Any substance taken internally that will promote sweating.

Diuretic: A medicine or herb that can cause an increase in the flow of urine.

Dyspepsia: Just a fancy way of saying indigestion.

Emmenagogue: Medicine or herb, taken internally, that will promote the flow of the menses.

Emollient: Substance that, when applied externally, will soften and soothe the skin.

Epithelium: Thin layer of cells forming a tissue that covers surfaces and lines hollow organs of the body.

Expectorant: A remedy that loosens phlegm, allowing it to be easily brought up and expectorated.

Febrifuge: A remedy that will reduce fever.

Herbarium: A collection of dried plants arranged systematically so that they can be easily studied.

Hygroscopic: Having the ability to attract and absorb moisture from the surrounding environment.

Jaundice: A diseased condition that causes the skin, eyes, and body fluids to turn a yellowish-green color. When the superstitious doctrine of signatures was in vogue, some herbalists tried to cure jaundice with yellow-flowered plants, while others insisted that red-flowered ones should be used to restore a healthy color. Both were wrong.

Jellies, jams, and jars: The best jars I have found for jellies and jams are the straight-sided, half-pint size that are usually called freezer jars. These can be sealed with regular, two-piece metal lids and require no messy paraffin. If the jelly or jam is cooked, it can be stored in any cupboard, but if it is the uncooked jam that can be made from many herbs mentioned in this book, it should be stored in the refrigerator if it is to be used within one month and in the freezer if it is to be kept longer. Because of the straight sides on these jars, the jelly or stiffly jellied jam can be unmolded so it can be served in a fancy dish, and these herbal delicacies deserve fancy dishes.

Lipase: An enzyme necessary to the proper digestion of fats.

Nephritis: Inflammation of the kidneys.

Nervine: An herb or medicine that will quiet nervousness or act as a tonic to nerve tissue. A relaxant or calmative.

Panicle: A loose, diversely branching flower cluster; a sort of compound raceme. Oats, reeds, and many other members of the grass family bear their flowers and seeds in panicles.

Pepper sauce: I had no idea this phrase would need defining, but several Yankees who looked over this manuscript had never heard of pepper sauce. It is no more than a bottle with a sprinkler top filled with tiny, very hot peppers pickled in vinegar. The peppers are not eaten, but the pepper-flavored vinegar is sprinkled over many kinds of food. When the supply runs low the bottle is merely refilled with fresh vinegar; the peppers are so powerful that they can be used for years. In the South, where I was raised, anyone who would serve green vegetables without having pepper sauce on the table would be considered a culinary heretic.

Petiole: The slender stalk by which a leaf is attached to a stem.

Pistillate: Adjective meaning the female part of the flower. Some plants have both the pistillate and staminate, or male and female, parts in the same flower, and such flowers are called "perfect." On others both kinds of flowers may be borne on the same plant, and on still others they are borne on separate plants. A pistil-packing flower is always a female.

Poultice: A soft, gooey mass, usually of crushed vegetable matter, applied to the surface of the body as a remedy for many disorders. Seldom used in modern medicine.

Raceme: A simple flower cluster having its flowers on nearly equal-length stalks along a stem, the lower flowers blooming first. The lily-of-the-valley bears its flowers on racemes.

Refrigerant: An old medical term for an internal medicine or herbal remedy that would cool the blood and reduce fever.

Restorative: A remedy or food that will get rid of that tired feeling.

Rheumatism: A sort of catch-all term that includes rheumatic fever, rheumatoid arthritis, and almost any pain and stiffness of the joints.

Rubefacient: A substance that will redden the surface of the skin or the lining of a hollow organ by attracting blood to that area.

Scurvy: The symptoms of an acute deficiency of vitamin C, characterized by swollen and bleeding gums, livid spots on the skin, and prostration. Formerly very common among sailors on long voyages.

Serrations: The sawlike teeth around the margins of some leaves.

Soporific: Anything that tends to induce sleep.

Spadix: A fleshy, more or less elongated spike that bears the minute flowers of some plants. In the Jack-in-the-pulpit the "Jack" is the spadix.

Spathe: A bract or hood enclosing the spadix. In Jack-in-the-pulpit the "pulpit" is the spathe.

Staminate: An adjective pertaining to the male, or pollen-bearing, part of a flower.

Stimulant: An herbal stimulant merely increases the activity of some part of the body, and not all stimulants bring a feeling of well-being. Stimulants must be carefully distinguished from narcotics, which often bring a feeling of euphoria by depressing certain nerve centers, causing us to temporarily forget our fears and woes.

Styptic: A substance that will check or stop bleeding. Most herbal styptics are strong astringents that stanch the flow of blood by shrinking the surrounding tissues, thus closing the exposed blood vessels.

Thoracic (Pertaining to the chest): An herb used to treat complaints of the lungs and bronchial tubes.

Tonic: Anything that gives strength or tone to the body. Bitter tonics achieve this by stimulating the flow of gastric juices, which increases the appetite, enabling the patient to consume more nourishing food. It is the food that restores strength, in this case.

Tubercle: A small, rounded projection or swelling.

Umbel: A flower cluster in which stalks of nearly equal length spring from a common center and form a flat or slightly curved surface.

Urethritis: Infection of the urethra, the duct by which urine is discharged from the bladder.

Vermifuge: A remedy that destroys parasitical intestinal worms and aids in expelling them.

Vitamin: An ill-defined term meaning a substance found in natural foodstuffs that is essential to growth or health. It seems certain that there are still many undiscovered vitamins that will be brought to our attention only when food processors refine them out of our diet and we begin to suffer. This is known as progress.

Vulnerary: An old-fashioned term for any herb used in treating battle wounds. Vulneraries were understandably popular when knights rode about slaying and wounding one another. Since most vulneraries are flowering plants, maybe the cliché, "When knighthood was in flower," has more meaning than we suspected.